Over 100 Chiropractors

Is your neck stiff when you get out of bed? As you go through your workday? When you make a meal? When you drive to the store? Stand in the line at the bank? If so, you need this book.

NECK PAIN, NECK PAIN
You Don't Want It, You Don't Need It

This book has been painstakingly researched and compiled
so that you never again have to suffer a
PAIN IN THE NECK!

Supported by the extensive experience of over 100 contributing chiropractic neck specialists, Dr. Fernandez has written the definitive manual for practical and proper neck maintenance.

Dr. Fernandez has been a chiropractor for over forty years. Among his specialties is the diagnosis and treatment of whiplash injuries and the care of neck injuries. In this regard, he became acutely aware that there was too little information available regarding comprehensive self-care of the neck.

Believing that people could prevent their neck problems if they only knew what to do, and with the enthusiastic support of over 100 chiropractors, Dr. Fernandez compiled this remarkable book.

All the information—the tips and techniques—presented in this ground-breaking book have resulted from tens of thousands of hours of service by devoted chiropractic neck-care specialists.

YOU WILL LEARN:

- The various postures, positions, and movements as well as household, recreational, and work activities that can cause neck pain.

- The household activities that place a strain on your neck. You will learn how to eliminate or modify some of these activities to reduce the chances of injuring your neck.

- The effects of automobiles and trucks on your neck … and how to reduce or eliminate the factors that cause these injuries.

- How to neck-proof your home and workplace—modify surfaces and activities to reduce the strains they place on your neck.

- How to strengthen your neck muscles. The stronger the muscles of your neck, the less neck problems you will have.

The practical advice of one of the most honored chiropractors in America and over 100 contributing chiropractic neck-care specialists can help you save your own neck!

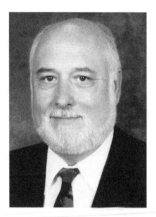

Peter G. Fernandez, D.C.

Paralyzed by polio from the waist down, barely able to breathe, and just seven years old, Peter Fernandez found his angel. She was Dr. Jeanette Hundley, a chiropractor in Fort Lauderdale, Florida. Defying what the other specialists had told Peter's mother, this angel said that he didn't have to be paralyzed. She was certain he could regain the use of his legs and lungs and become an active and productive adult.

Ten years after receiving the care of this wonderful chiropractor and determined to follow in his angel's footsteps, Peter attended his first class at chiropractic college at the age of 17. Eager to begin helping others to healthier, happier, and more productive lives, he studied chiropractic principles year-round, not taking summers off. Just three years later, he became Dr. Peter Fernandez. By the age of 21, he was a practicing chiropractor, devoted to continuing to learn as much as he could in order to provide his patients with the best possible care.

For the next 20 years, Dr. Fernandez practiced chiropractic with a passion, always working to expand and improve his skills, his efforts earning him numerous post-graduate honors. With happy patients and a flourishing practice, he grew to have five associates practicing with him in his clinic in St. Petersburg, Florida, plus a chain of 12 chiropractic clinics throughout the United States, all using his practice methods of fast relief for neck and back pain, and teaching patients how to care for and cure their neck and back problems.

An active member of his profession, he became president of his local chiropractic society, then president of the prestigious Florida Chiropractic Association and the chairman of the Eastern division of the Chiropractic Knights of the Round Table, one of the chiropractic profession's most honored societies. In 1986, he was appointed the national chiropractic director of Doctors with a Heart, the world's largest doctor-sponsored charity. In 1991, Dr. Fernandez was recognized for his work and commitment to Doctors with a Heart and was appointed national chairman by the founder, Dr. Duane Schmidt. He has remained chairman of Doctors with a Heart and gladly dedicates his time to promoting the charity, which provides free healthcare services to those patients who can't otherwise afford it.

Having worked so hard to acquire the knowledge and skills that allowed him to reach and exceed his professional goals, he realized that if more chiropractors knew what he knew, more patients would get well and more lives would be improved. Twenty-five years later, he continues to teach new doctors how to establish successful practices and established doctors how to be more effective. Dr. Fernandez has taught more than 10,000 chiropractors and almost 20,000 support personnel. He has also written 20 books, 50 manuals, and more than 100 published articles on the practice of chiropractic.

Dr. Fernandez specializes in the care of neck injuries, in the diagnosis and treatment of whiplash injuries as well as disc problems in the lower back and sciatica.

NECK PAIN
NECK PAIN
You Don't Want It, You Don't Need It

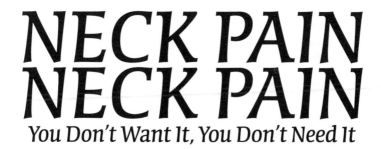

NECK PAIN NECK PAIN
You Don't Want It, You Don't Need It

The Neck Pain Prevention
Secrets of Over 100 Chiropractors

Peter G. Fernandez, D.C.

FERNANDEZ PRESS • SEMINOLE, FL

Neck Pain, Neck Pain: You Don't Want It, You Don't Need It

©2007 by Dr. Peter Fernandez

Fernandez Press
10733 57th Avenue, North
Seminole, FL 33772
(800) 882-4476/(727) 392-0489 fax
www.FernandezPress.com
info@FernandezPress.com

This book is for educational purposes. It is not intended as a substitute for medical advice. Please consult a qualified health care professional for individual health and medical advice. Neither the publisher nor the author shall have any responsibility for any adverse effects arising directly or indirectly as a result of the information provided in this book.

Publishers Cataloguing-in-Publication

Fernandez, Peter G.

    Neck pain, neck pain : you don't want it, you don't need it / Peter G.
    Fernandez. -- Seminole, FL : Fernandez Press, 2007.

       p. ; cm.
      ISBN-13: 978-0-9789249-5-9
      ISBN-10: 0-9789249-5-9
      "The neck pain prevention secrets of over 100 chiropractors."--
    Cover.
      Includes index.

      1. Neck pain. 2. Neck pain--Prevention. 3. Neck pain--Exercise
    therapy. 4. Neck--Care and hygiene. 5. Consumer education.
    I. Title.

RD763 .F47 2007   2006935253
617.5/3--dc22   0701

Book and cover designer: Pamela Terry, Opus 1 Design
www.Opus1design.com
Cover Photo: Photos.com
Editor: Brookes Nohlgren
Book Consultant: Ellen Reid, www.bookshep.com

Printed in the United States of America on acid-free paper

DEDICATION

I dedicate this book to my wonderful wife, Cathy, without whose encouragement and understanding this work would not have been possible. Thank you for giving up your husband for the thousands of hours it took to write this book.

And, to the many chiropractic neck specialists who unselfishly contributed their time and expertise to the content of this book ... I thank you and dedicate this book to you.

It is also with great appreciation that I acknowledge the professional contribution and empowering support and encouragement I received from my forever friend and colleague, Dr. R. Wayne Pitts. Growing up in this profession together, Wayne and I shared in countless achievements and challenges. Though not brothers by blood, we became brothers by heart. Sadly, Wayne passed away shortly before this book went to press. However, his generous and caring spirit continues to touch people, including those who will achieve a life free from neck pain by following the expert advice given in this book. Thank you, friend.

ACKNOWLEDGMENTS

Obviously, no one person could assemble a book of this magnitude. I've had a lot of help and would like to acknowledge all of the people who made this book possible.

Thank you … thank you … thank you … to the 100-plus doctors who gave their time and expertise to this book. And thank you on behalf of the thousands of readers who will find in this book the help they need.

Susie Hensley, my assistant for over fifteen years, who spent hundreds of hours typing, retyping, making suggestions and additions … I thank you.

To Valerie Carbonneau, whose writing skills astonish me. Thanks for adding your thoughts, ideas, writing and organizational skills to this endeavor. Your skills make me look much better.

To Ellen Reid, my "book shepherd" … thanks for guiding me through the maze of technicalities to complete this book. Your help was invaluable.

Brookes Nohlgren and Laren Bright, my superb editors … thanks for your help. No matter how skilled an author is, it's professional editors who assure a book's reader the most enjoyable reading experience, by repositioning content for maximum continuity, deleting redundancies, and correcting spelling and punctuation. To both of my editors, my heartfelt thanks.

Larry Headley is not only a talented illustrator, he must also be the most patient individual in the world. This book contains 471 illustrations, all of which were hand-drawn, and re-drawn, at least four or five times. Thanks, Larry, for sticking with me throughout this project.

And, last but not least, my thanks to Pamela Terry, my book cover designer and book layout expert. The beautiful cover, the visual appeal of each page, and the artful placement of the illustrations are all a result of her genius.

To all of you … THANK YOU!

COMPILATION DISCLAIMER

This book is a compilation of the neck pain prevention suggestions received from over one hundred doctors of chiropractic. These doctors have represented that the information given is true, accurate, and theirs to provide.

This book serves as an information resource, not medical advice. The reader remains solely liable for determining whether ideas contained in this book are appropriate for the reader.

Table of Contents

Introduction: How to Use This Book

I congratulate you for taking time out of your busy schedule to learn how to prevent neck problems. This book is a self-help survival manual for people who want to have a healthy, strong, pain-free neck. After forty-five years of taking care of patients with neck pain, I have found that the most proactive way to deal with neck problems is to find out what is causing the neck pain and then stop doing those activities or behaviors. Most neck pain is preventable, that is, *if* you have the knowledge to prevent it. This book will give you that knowledge.

You will discover which postures, positions, and movements as well as which household, recreational, and work activities can cause neck pain. You will also learn how to make your environment safer for your neck, or more **neck-friendly,** by using the principles of ergonomics.

ERGONOMICS

The word *ergonomics* describes the relationship of the human body to its environment (e.g., tools, counter heights, etc.). As you know, human beings come in many sizes—some tall, some short, some with long torsos, others with short arms, others with long legs, and so on. And, most surfaces that we use to play, work, or sit do not match our individual body sizes and shapes. Therefore, in order for us to be comfortable with our environments, the surfaces and chairs on which we work or play have to be adjusted to our bodies, or our bodies will adjust to these surfaces.

Neck-ergonomics is the relationship of your neck to its environment. For example, does your neck have to bend to read a document, watch TV, or drive a vehicle? When you use correct neck-ergonomics, you will be able to conduct your daily activities without hurting your neck.

NECK-PROOFING

You can adapt your environment to your body by modifying anything that may cause a neck strain or injury. For example, you can lubricate doors, drawers, and windows and store items at specific heights that allow you to reach for them without bending your neck.

However, no matter how diligently you try to maintain good posture, an environment that is not adjusted to fit your body type (i.e., height, weight, etc.) will continue to force *you* to fit *it*, and the results will be progressively poor posture. Adjusting your environment to your body type to achieve and maintain a healthy positive posture, or you to it, is called **neck-proofing.** Neck-proofing will greatly reduce your chances of experiencing **neck-attacks,** or damage to your neck.

NECK-CONSCIOUSNESS

There are many things you can do at home and work to prevent neck injuries. Learn how to neck-proof your environment by following the instructions in this book, and you will reduce your chances of having neck problems. The awareness of which movements, postures, and activities cause neck problems and knowing how to modify your environment to avoid neck pain is called **neck-consciousness**. The more neck-conscious you become by reading this book, the better care you can take of your neck and the less likely it will be that a neck problem will occur.

NECK-INSTRUCTIONS

Throughout the chapter on exercising (Chapter 16), you will notice "doctor instructions." I hope that you will take this book to your chiropractor and have him or her check off the specific exercises that he or she feels are appropriate for you to do, or not do. For example, your doctor may prescribe certain exercises to strengthen your neck, yet he or she may specifically tell you not to do other exercises that may antagonize an injury you already have.

NECK-APPLIANCES AND NECK-AIDS

Also throughout this book you will find recommendations for **neck-appliances** and **neck-aids**, such as neck pillows, rolls, and exercise devices, that can help keep your neck healthy. I recommend that you have your chiropractor prescribe those neck-aids and neck-appliances he or she feels will aid *your* neck. For your convenience, I have followed each item mentioned with a product number (e.g., [18]) and have also included a complete list of these items in numeric order on page 269. You may purchase these products from your family chiropractor or from the Neck and Back Products store at *www.NeckAndBackProducts.com* or by calling 1-800-882-4476. This company is a great source for neck-care aids and appliances, including those hard-to-find items.

NECK-CARE

Throughout this book you will be told to consult a chiropractor. Chiropractors treat the majority of neck injuries. Over 100 of these neck-care specialists have contributed to the writing of this book and are honored in the Appendix.

Let this book be your guide to better neck health and greater neck comfort. Read it more than once. Develop neck-consciousness, then follow the guidelines of this book to a stronger, healthier neck.

WHAT YOU WILL LEARN

SECTION ONE: THE NECK AND BACK CONNECTION

The first section of this book contains two chapters.

Chapter 1 teaches you the vital structures of a healthy spine.

Chapter 2 reveals how posture affects your neck—poor posture is one of the biggest causes of neck problems.

SECTION TWO: REDUCING NECK STRAINS IN DAILY LIFE

The second section of this book details the many ways we as human beings place strains upon our neck. The more you strain your neck the more neck problems you will have. And, similarly, the more you can reduce the strains to your neck, the better neck health you will enjoy.

Chapter 3 describes the bodily movements and positions that strain your neck and what you can do to modify these activities for better neck health.

Chapter 4 discusses how to maintain proper posture while sleeping. Believe it or not, many people produce an eight-hour strain to their neck every night while sleeping. This chapter explains the type of pillows and bedding you can use to maintain proper posture while sleeping and describes the correct sleeping postures.

Chapter 5 describes the household activities that place a strain on your neck. You will learn how to eliminate or modify some of these activities to reduce the chances of injuring your neck.

Chapter 6 describes how typical bathing, washing, shaving, and dressing activities can strain your neck muscles and provides instructions on how to modify these activities in order to not strain your neck.

Chapter 7 describes many of the activities mothers and fathers perform in raising their children—carrying, lifting, changing diapers, placing children in automobiles, and so on—and explains how, if done improperly, these activities may injure your neck. Then, you will learn how to do these activities in a neck-friendly manner.

Chapter 8 discusses the negative effects driving and riding in automobiles and trucks have on your neck. Certain body positions can cause strains, and the vibrations from the vehicles can injure the discs of your neck. In this chapter you will learn how to reduce or eliminate the factors that cause these injuries.

Chapter 9 discusses the recreational activities we enjoy; some are good, producing very little strain to the neck, and some are bad, producing a lot of neck strain.

Chapter 10 describes the stresses that long-distance traveling can place on your neck and how to reduce or eliminate these stresses.

Chapter 11 reveals the strenuous activities that occasionally we all must do that cause serious injury to the neck. You will learn how to minimize the injuries that can be caused by these types of activities.

SECTION THREE: NECK-PROOFING YOUR WORLD

Section Three will show you how to maintain correct posture at home, work, and play, and how to neck-proof your environment so that your environment (i.e., work and play surfaces, chairs, computers, etc.) does not hurt your neck. Improper posture is one of the main causes of neck strain. Changing the way you stand, sit, or lie down or changing your environment to fit your body will reduce neck strain caused by poor posture.

Chapter 12 describes how to modify your household surfaces and activities to reduce strains to your neck.

Chapter 13 teaches you how to modify your vehicle to reduce the vibrations that damage the discs of your neck as well as how to minimize the strains your vehicle places on your neck in other ways.

Chapter 14 describes how to neck-proof your workplace when you have a sitting occupation. This chapter includes how to modify your work surfaces, chair, and desk to fit your body instead of forcing your body to fit them.

Chapter 15 describes neck-proofing your workplace when you have a standing occupation. This chapter teaches you how to modify your standing work surfaces, chairs, computers, and so on to match your height and body type, reducing the stress to your neck produced by a bad fit between you and your work environment.

SECTION FOUR: CREATING A STRONG NECK

Section Four teaches you how to strengthen your neck. Once you have neck-proofed your environment and eliminated everything that produces neck strains, you can further reduce the chances of hurting your neck by strengthening your neck muscles. The stronger the muscles of your neck, the fewer neck problems you will have.

Chapter 16 describes how to effectively stretch and strengthen your neck, shoulder, and mid back muscles.

APPENDIX: RESOURCES

The Appendix contains resources for greater neck health. It includes a convenient numerical listing of the neck-aids and neck-appliances mentioned in this book. These products, including those hard-to-find items, are available through your chiropractor or by contacting the Neck and Back Products store at *www.NeckAndBackProducts.com* or 1-800-882-4476.

This section also acknowledges the many fine neck specialist chiropractors who devoted so much of their time contributing to the writing of this book and provides you with their contact information. If you have any questions regarding the recommendations in this book, these contributing authors will be happy to help you.

After reading this book, you will have an abundance of **neck-smarts.** Acting on these will help ensure that you have a healthy, pain-free neck!

Section One:

The Neck and Back Connection

1

Understanding Your Spine

To maintain a healthy, strong neck that is pain free, you must first understand your neck—what it is made of, how it works, and how it gets injured. In this chapter, you will get a brief lesson about the anatomy of your spine and neck and a short explanation of the most common causes of neck problems.

Spinal Anatomy

Your spinal column is an engineering marvel. This strong, bony structure supports the weight of your head and body. It also serves as the main attachment for your neck and back muscles. It is flexible, yet provides protection for your spinal cord and nerves that carry messages from your brain to the rest of your body. And it does all of these jobs simultaneously.

If you were to look at your spine from the back, you would see that the spinal bones **(vertebrae)** are in the center. The vertebrae are not close to the skin, as one might imagine; rather, they are two inches below the skin and stacked one on top of the other from the top of your pelvis to the bottom of your skull. This long, flexible column of bones carries both the weight of your head—which is slightly heavier than a gallon of milk—and that of your upper body.

If you were to look at your body from the side, you would see four curves—two forward-bending curves, one in your neck and the other in your lower back, and two backward-bending curves, one in your mid back and one in your pelvic area. These opposing curves absorb the shocks of daily living.

VERTEBRAE

You have twenty-four vertebrae—seven in the **cervical** (neck) area, twelve in the **thoracic** (chest) area, and five in the **lumbar** (lower back) area. When you were a child, there were also five vertebrae in your pelvic area, which fused together as an adult to form the **sacrum.** The three small bones at the bottom of the sacrum make up the tailbone **(coccyx).**

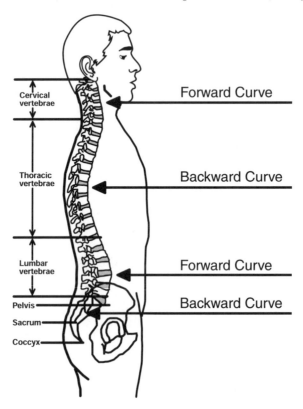

Cervical vertebrae

Forward Curve

Thoracic vertebrae

Backward Curve

Lumbar vertebrae

Forward Curve

Pelvis

Backward Curve

Sacrum

Coccyx

Normal Curves of Spine

Most vertebrae consist of a thick, strong, weight-bearing portion at the front of each vertebra and a ring of bone at the back of each vertebra that surrounds the spinal cord. The opening in the ring is called the **spinal canal.** Attached to the middle of each ring are four upward and downward bony projections that create four joints that interlock each vertebra with the vertebrae above and below. These are your **facet joints,** which are approximately the size of your finger joints. They allow restricted forward, backward, sideways, and rotational movements, and they also serve as attachments for muscles. A bony projection called a **spinous process** extends directly back from the ring of bone. This is the bump you notice when you feel the back of your neck. Two other bony projections, called **transverse processes,** extend off the sides of the ring. The spinous processes and transverse processes provide attachments for the muscles that control spinal motion.

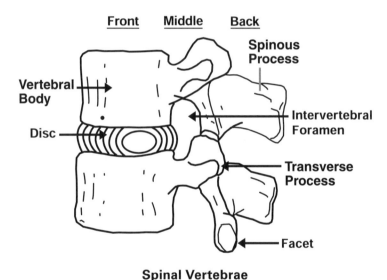

Spinal Vertebrae

Spinal vertebrae have different characteristics depending on their location. The cervical (neck) vertebrae are the smallest because they support the least weight. The upper cervical vertebrae are shaped differently to allow for rotation of the head and neck, while the bodies of the remaining cervical vertebrae have "u" shaped joints, called **Luschka joints,** which limit sideways bending and rotation of the neck. Your thoracic (chest) vertebrae are larger than the cervical vertebrae and have dish-shaped attachments for the ribs. The lumbar (lower back) vertebrae are the largest because they carry all the weight of the body above the waist.

MUSCLES

The portion of your spine that makes up your neck contains dozens of **muscles** that contract and relax every time you move your head—which for most people happens approximately 3,000 to 4,000 times a day on average. The neck muscles perform a very difficult engineering feat, similar to balancing a wobbling bowling ball on top of a finger. It is no wonder they get tired and weak.

LIGAMENTS

The vertebrae are held in place by tough, fibrous bands of tissue called **ligaments,** which surround the spine. The ligaments' main function is to hold the vertebrae together. They provide stability while allowing you to bend and twist within safe ranges.

INTERVERTEBRAL DISCS

Between the spinal vertebrae (except the top two), there are flat, semi-hard ligaments called **intervertebral discs.** These discs make up one-fourth of the length of the spinal column. Each disc binds two vertebrae together. The discs are made of tough, fibrous material surrounding a jelly-like center. This jelly-like center is about 80 percent water. Bearing weight compresses the discs during the day, forcing out the water, which accounts for a daily height loss of one-half to one inch. As the spine rests at night, no longer bearing weight, the discs reabsorb the water and height is restored.

SPINAL CORD

Your **spinal cord** is a pliable column of nerve tissue extending from the bottom of your brain to your second lumbar vertebra, which is at the level of your belt line. On average, it is about seventeen inches long and the width of your little finger. It lies protected within the spinal canal.

SPINAL NERVES

Branches of nerves **(spinal nerves)** exit the spinal cord between both sides of each vertebra. The nerves that leave the spinal cord in the upper neck become the nerves of the neck and head. The nerves that leave the spinal cord in the lower neck become the nerves of the arms and hands. The nerves that leave the spinal cord in the lower back form the nerves going down the legs.

The majority of the signals to and from your brain are carried through the spinal cord and its nerves. One set of nerves reports your bodily functions and sensations of touch, heat, cold, pain, position, and movement. Another set of nerves directs your muscles to move and your body functions to change. Additional nerves leave the spinal cord and go to the organs and blood vessels of the body. For each sensation and body function, there is a different set of nerves carrying the messages to and from your brain. When the spinal cord is injured, messages cannot get through from the body to the brain, and vice versa. Depending on where the cord is hurt, and how much damage is done, the injury can mean partial or complete paralysis, or even death.

Spinal Motion

The motion of your neck is quite different from that of the rest of your spine. Nearly half of your neck movement occurs at the upper two cervical vertebrae, immediately below your skull, where there are no facet or Luschka joints to limit rotational movement. Because this area is highly movable, it is very vulnerable to injury. After all, what moves a lot can be moved too far.

The remaining vertebrae in your neck have adequate forward and backward motion, but are severely restricted in rotational motion because the facet and Luschka joints allow your spinal bones to lean to the side or rotate only so far before acting as a doorstop. No further movement will be allowed in either direction. To illustrate how your facet and Luschka joints work, look as far to the left or to the right as you can. You will notice that your neck will only rotate so far, and then it stops. The facet and Luschka joints are preventing your neck from moving too far.

The Primary Causes of Neck Pain

SPINAL MISALIGNMENT

When vertebrae are out of their proper alignment, the result is improper motion—the number one reason for neck discomfort and pain. To understand this better, first consider the anatomy of the human neck—a thin, highly mobile column of bones, held together only by ligaments and discs, that balances a heavy head. Then consider the numerous blows suffered to a person's head and neck throughout a lifetime. As the father of seven children, whom I have watched fall—out of high chairs, off of couches, and out of trees—play football, wrestle, and fight, I wonder how they did not misalign their spines more. Unfortunately, the majority of people <u>do</u> misalign their necks when they are young and, not knowing that they have done so, never have their necks properly realigned by a chiropractor. The longer a vertebra is out of alignment, the further the restraining ligaments stretch, the more arthritis will occur in that joint, and the more difficult it will be to realign the vertebra.

MUSCLE WEAKNESS

Chapter 16 describes how to strengthen the muscles of your neck. This is crucial to a healthy neck because the stronger the neck muscles, the less likely injuries to the neck are to occur. When neck muscles are weak, they are not able to hold the head or neck in the correct, upright posture. Neck muscles that have lost strength will allow the neck vertebrae to slip out of alignment. The weaker the neck muscles, the worse neck posture becomes. Therefore, anyone wanting a pain-free, problem-free neck should not only have a properly aligned neck, but also strong neck muscles to support it.

STRUCTURAL DISORDERS OF THE SPINE

Prolonged improper posture will many times misalign or malform entire sections of the spine. The **"widow's hump"** or **"Dowagers hump"** deformity is an example. The upper and mid back become hunched as a result of a **head-forward posture,** when the head is carried forward of the rest of the spine. The weight of the head pushing forward and down forces the upper and mid back to become rounded. The lower back then sags forward in an attempt to maintain balance.

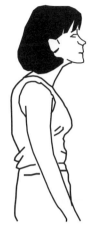
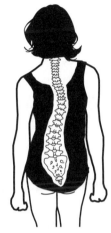

Dowager's Hump   **Scoliosis**

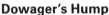

Scoliosis is another structural deformity of the spine. This is when the curves of the spine are exaggerated to the side, backward or forward, or a combination of these. This condition predominantly affects adolescent or teenage children, and it affects females eight times as often as males. A temporary scoliosis can be found immediately after an injury, as the spine is pulled into an abnormal curvature by muscle spasms. Once the muscle spasms are relieved, however, the spine will usually return to its original position.

When a structural disorder such as scoliosis occurs, it produces excessive strain on certain areas of the spine, misaligning them. The resulting changes in weight bearing can lead to excessive strain on the hips, eventually causing arthritis and degeneration of the hip joints. Because this deformity constantly pulls the spine in unhealthy directions, this type of misalignment is difficult to correct. Fortunately, however, it is correctable most of the time.

INJURIES

A significant percentage of misalignments of the neck are caused by injury, which can severely damage fragile neck structures. Neck vertebrae can be broken, dented, or crushed. Whiplash injuries from automobile accidents are a primary reason people seek chiropractic care. Sports and falls also contribute greatly to neck injuries. Any injury to the neck can cause serious problems and predispose the injured person to neck pain as well as degenerative arthritis in the future.

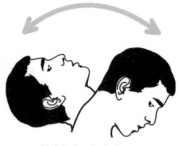

Whiplash Injury

STRAINS AND SPRAINS

Two primary causes of neck pain, and a major focus of this book, are strains and sprains. When a *muscle* or *tendon* is stretched or torn, it is called a **strain.** A **sprain** is when *ligaments* or *discs* are stretched, ripped, or ruptured.

Strains and sprains occur in varying degrees. A muscle can be suddenly ripped (strain). This occurs quite often in athletes who overexert a muscle. Ligaments can also be ripped by a sudden effort (sprain). For example, an individual who suddenly twists his or her ankle and rips (partially or completely) the ligaments that hold the ankle together suffers a sprain.

Muscles can be strained to a lesser degree by repetitiously doing a one-sided activity over a long period of time. Continuously pulling on the muscles on one side of your neck, such as when working or reading in a bent-over posture, stretches them little by little and ultimately injures the muscles. The prolonged bending of your head and neck forward stretches your neck muscles, which weakens them and allows your vertebrae to shift out of alignment. Continued stretching of these muscles can cause them to fray and possibly rip over time. The same pattern of overstretching, fraying, and then ripping can also occur with ligaments. A minor repetitious sprain may lead to a more serious sprain, and ultimately to a rupture of the ligaments.

Why are straining and spraining such serious problems? Because muscles are responsible for moving bones and supporting proper posture. When spinal muscles become strained, the spine sags in one direction, causing discomfort and pain and misaligning vertebrae that can then cause pressure on the nerves that go from the spine to all other parts of the body. Pressure on nerves can hurt and even become incapacitating!

Ligaments hold bones together. If a spinal ligament is stretched or ripped (a sprain), vertebrae will misalign, resulting in irritated nerves and spinal problems. Therefore, preventing strains and sprains of the neck and back muscles is paramount for avoiding more serious neck problems.

VIBRATION

The discs of your spine are very susceptible to the effects of micro-traumas (mini-shocks). Excessive riding in a vehicle, some types of dancing, jogging, horseback riding, riding dirt bikes, water skiing, and riding in boats all produce vibrations that can injure your spinal discs and lead to arthritis. Excessive vibration to a weakened spine can actually shake spinal vertebrae out of alignment, producing pain. As a side note, to help prevent vibrational injuries, drink adequate amounts of water throughout the day.

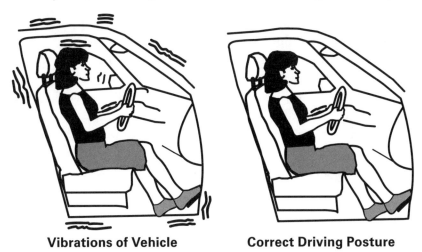

Vibrations of Vehicle　　　　**Correct Driving Posture**

DISEASE PROCESSES

Tumors, infections, and other disease processes in the neck area can also affect the structures of your neck. Fortunately, such neck conditions are very rare. One common disease that affects the neck is **degenerative**

osteoarthritis, which causes the vertebrae, discs, and spinal joints to wear down prematurely. This type of osteoarthritis is not usually the cause of neck pain but a secondary effect of other problems. As mentioned, the primary causes of neck pain are spinal misalignments, muscle weakness, injuries, muscle strains, and ligament sprains.

DRAFTS OF AIR

Drafts of air continually hitting your neck can cause your neck muscles to tighten and become spastic, which may pull your vertebrae out of place. This is a major cause of Torticollis (Wry Neck), a very painful twisting and tilting of the neck to the side.

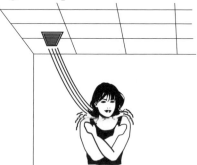

Avoid Drafts on Neck

MENTAL STRESS

In addition to strains, sprains, diseases, and bodily injuries, mental stress can create neck pain. If you are angry, your muscles may tense without your realizing it. The longer the tension lasts, the more likely your muscles will harden into painful knots.

Whether caused by an injury, continuous poor posture, strains, sprains, or an infection, neck pain is something that should be taken seriously. Even minimal pain means that something is wrong and needs to be fixed. If it is not fixed, it will likely get worse. As a supplement to professional help or as a guide to self-treatment, this book will show you how to avoid injuring your neck, how to strengthen it, and how to create an environment that helps to prevent neck pain.

2

Posture and a Pain-Free Neck

G ood posture is one of the best-kept secrets of good health. It is as important as eating, sleeping, and exercising properly. When you use correct posture, the bones of your spine distribute the weight of your body properly. Then, the muscles and ligaments of your spine are required to do only minimal work to support you. Good posture keeps your organs hanging in their proper positions, creates deeper breathing, and puts less stress on your heart.

Neck problems rarely are caused by a single injury, even though they can be, such as with a whiplash, a blow, or an impact. More often than not, neck pain is the result of *neck strains caused by poor posture* sustained over a long period of time from unhealthy daily working and living habits. It has been estimated that 80 percent of all neck and back pain is caused by tight, strained muscles resulting from years of poor posture. For that reason, maintaining correct posture in your daily activities is a main focus of this book.

The Four Curves

The key to proper posture is maintaining the four curves of your spine, whether you are standing, sitting, or lying down. These curves give your spine a springing action—like a shock absorber—which protects it from daily jolts and jars. Too little of a curve in your neck or lower back will cause your vertebrae to jam against each other and become misaligned. These abnormal neck curves will cause a pinching of the intervertebral discs, which will degenerate the discs, producing arthritis and placing pressure on the nerves. The result is swelling, spasms, and pain. Too much of a curve in the neck forces the weight of the head to be carried on the facets of the back portion of your neck instead of on the front of the spinal bones, which is the weight-bearing portion of your vertebrae. The more you keep the curves of your neck and back properly aligned, the less pain you will have and the healthier you will be.

The Problem with Poor Posture

Improper posture stretches the spinal ligaments out of shape, allowing the curves of the spine to straighten or reverse, and ultimately causing misaligned vertebrae, a misaligned skull, nerve problems, and pain. Reversed spinal curves can also occur from repetitive physical activity, muscles pulling too tightly, a whiplash injury, and slack spinal muscles or ligaments.

Among the many ill effects of poor posture are compression of the nerves that extend from the neck to the top of the head, which produces headaches, and compression or stretching of the nerves that course down the arms and legs, which produces pain, paresthesias (numbness, tingling, electric-like feelings, etc.), and difficulty breathing. And, difficult breathing can start a dangerous "snowball" effect. For example, sleep apnea studies have concluded that when a person cannot breathe properly it raises his or her blood pressure, which in turn stresses the heart.

The ill effects that poor posture can have on breathing can best be illustrated by doing the following exercise. Sit totally erect with your head up, and then inhale deeply. Then hang your head forward about three inches with your chin level to the ground and, once again, inhale deeply. You will notice that you are not able to take as deep a breath with your head held forward as you can when sitting erect.

Once posture sags, the neck becomes vulnerable, and just one sudden stressful activity or twist of the neck can produce pain or injury.

Besides the physical problems produced by poor posture, the visual aesthetics (i.e., how it looks) have to be considered. Poor posture looks horrible! Slouching gives the impression that a person lacks self-confidence.

Movie stars, models, and athletes all stand up straight, walk straight, and look great. What kind of impression do you want to make?

The Causes of Poor Posture

Human beings are creatures of habit. We form our habits often without realizing it, and then we are owned by them. Before long, we simply adjust our lives to maintain them. Our bodies are the same way. If you have negative posture habits, your body will adjust its comfort level to accommodate the postures you most often assume. Take, for example, someone whose job requires his or her head to be bent forward all day. Pretty soon, this posture tires out the individual's neck muscles and they become slack. The person's head and neck are now hanging forward on the neck ligaments, producing an ache or other pain. Soon, the individual will have to slouch to relieve the discomfort. The slouching makes the posture worse, producing more discomfort and thus more slouching to relieve that discomfort. It becomes a vicious cycle.

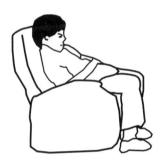

Avoid Slouching

Slouching exhausts your muscles and stretches your ligaments, allowing your normal spinal curves to first straighten and then reverse, producing aches and pains. Then, once the curves of your spine are straightened or reversed, you will slouch more to ease the discomfort and fatigue in your muscles, stretching your ligaments further, and producing more aches and pains. You now have a structural disorder that perpetuates your pain and the reversal of your spinal curves.

So, you can see why slouching is so bad even though it feels so good! Slouching is the body's attempt to slacken and relax muscles to relieve the discomfort of muscle strain. But, in fact, slouching stretches the muscles, causing them to tire and then hurt more. You sit in your favorite overstuffed chair to rest your body. But that same chair may force you to round your lower back, which forces your neck to round in the wrong direction. If you stay in that position for a while, your lower back and neck will start to hurt.

The only cure for slouching is to *eliminate the need to slouch*. If you are sitting or standing with correct posture, your body weight is correctly distributed on the portion of the spinal bones designed to support it. With the weight properly supported, there is no need to slouch. Your muscles can then relax, reducing the strain on them.

People begin to slouch for different reasons. Adolescence is most commonly when people develop poor posture. A teenager striving for individualism may slouch in an attempt to be "cool" or simply to defy his or her parents' request to "quit slouching and stand up straight." Some teenagers think going against an adult's directive is doing their "own thing." It is also during adolescence that many bodily changes occur, causing some young people to want to just blend into the scenery and go unnoticed. By slouching, they feel as though they are making themselves as small and invisible as possible. And sometimes young women, feeling self-conscious that they are too tall, assume a slumped forward posture to reduce their height. Other young women become embarrassed when they start to develop breasts and thus round their shoulders to hide their development.

Some postural problems result from a congenital abnormality, such as being born with one leg shorter than the other. This type of defect can easily lead to scoliosis (an excessive curving of the spine). Postural abnormalities, such as scoliosis, though not always correctable, can certainly be improved.

Spinal misalignments—caused by incidents such as car accidents, falls, contact sports, or children playing rough with one another—also can produce abnormal spinal curves that may cause shoulder heights to differ, a head-forward posture, or some other major postural problem. These types of postural problems are more difficult to correct and usually require the care of a chiropractor. They also require the complete and consistent cooperation of the person suffering from the condition.

Other causes of poor posture include inadequate sleeping support, unhealthy occupational positions, and poorly designed home and work surfaces. For example, children often spend many hours at a time playing video games and usually assume poor posture while doing so. Repeatedly sitting in an unhealthy position for long periods of time erodes a person's overall posture. And the longer a person uses poor posture, the more permanent it will likely become. The brain gradually interprets the posture

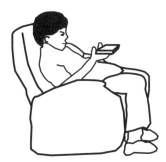

**Slouching While
Playing Games**

in which you spend the most time as "normal," and it will attempt to keep the body in this newest (actually abnormal) position.

So, why do people not improve their posture once they have survived adolescence? Because, as with any unhealthy habit, to stop slouching takes work and a conscious effort. But, if you understand the vital role that good posture plays in your physical and emotional well-being, you will be more motivated to do what it takes to stop the debilitating slouching cycle and correct your posture.

The Head-Forward Posture

The head-forward posture is a special type of incorrect posture. Not only is it the most common postural problem—suffered by approximately 66 percent of Americans—it is also the most serious. Sometimes, for various reasons, people carry their head not directly over their chest, but inches forward. This starts a dangerous chain reaction.

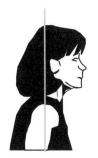

**Head-Forward
Posture**

The head weighs approximately twelve pounds, or slightly more than a gallon of milk. The human body was designed to have the head resting directly over the shoulders and rib cage. When the head is in this position, very little weight pushes down on the ligaments and muscles of the neck. Instead, the weight is carried by the bones of the neck. When looking at someone's posture from the side, for each inch that his or her head is forward of the center of the rib cage the downward pressure caused by the weight of the head increases by ten pounds. So, by being just three inches forward of its normal position, your head creates thirty pounds of additional pressure on your neck. The further forward you hold your head, the more your neck and upper back muscles have to work to keep your head up. In fact, when your head is held forward more than one inch, the muscles at the back of your neck automatically tighten with the same tension as an archer's bowstring in their attempt to bring your head back to its normal upright position. Placing this amount of tension on your neck muscles usually results in tension headaches, pain between your shoulder blades, and a restricted range of motion.

To demonstrate this effect, hold a gallon of milk close to your chest. You will likely be able to hold it there indefinitely. Now hold it three to four inches in front of you. Before long, your muscles will begin to ache from attempting to hold the milk. The muscles will become weak and exhausted, and the gallon of milk will sag, just like a person's head sags when in a head-forward posture.

Once the neck muscles become exhausted in their attempt to hold the head up, they begin to hurt and can no longer support the neck and head, and the body loses its main support for good posture. The body then transfers its postural support from the vertebrae to the ligaments of the spine. The spinal ligaments now have to support the weight of the head—which they were not designed to do. The ligaments soon become overstretched, causing chronic neck pain, upper back pain, stiffness, and fatigue. And once this process starts, if left uncorrected, it almost always gets worse.

When you have a head-forward posture, the muscles at the back of your neck become stretched and then tight. The muscles in the front of your neck shorten because they are not being used very much. Unfortunately, those stretched and tightened muscles at the back of your neck and upper back become responsible for holding up your head and neck.

In fact, when you have a head-forward posture, most of the work of holding your head up falls on the "pain in the neck" **trapezius muscle.** This muscle is large and diamond-shaped and runs from the bottom of your skull out to both shoulders and then down to your mid back. When your head hangs forward and down, the upper part of the trapezius muscle is placed under a tremendous strain in its attempt to hold up the (very heavy) head. When the head-forward posture lasts for a period of time, the trapezius muscle becomes tightened, thickened, and stiff, and the upper back becomes more rounded. The nerves that exit the bottom of the neck and go into the arms and hands become stretched and, many times, squeezed. The result is muscle tension, recurring neck pain, upper back pain, numbness or tingling in the arms and hands, chronic headaches, and

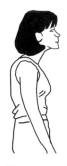

Dowager's Hump

an undesirable appearance of the upper back called a "widow's hump" or "Dowager's hump."

Individuals with a head-forward posture lose much of the rotational capacity of their neck. Most motions of the neck are coupled, meaning the neck moves in two directions at the same time. For example, you can turn your neck and look upward at the same time. With a head-forward posture, 25 to 50 percent of all coupled motion of the neck is eliminated. This results in a permanently stiffer neck.

To illustrate this loss, turn your head as far as you can to the left and right. Next, push your head three inches forward and again turn your head as far as you can in each direction. You will notice that, when your head is forward, you are no longer able to turn it as far as you could when it was in its correct position. Thus the neck becomes stiffer, and whenever the neck becomes stiffer there is a decrease in the stimulation of special sensing devices in the neck called mechanoreceptors. These mechanoreceptors send messages to the brain centers that control balance and the production of endorphins, the body's natural painkiller. With de-

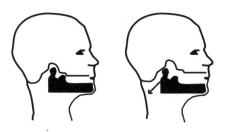

Misalignment of Jaw

creased mechanoreceptor stimulation, we feel pain more easily; therefore, any pain is amplified.

Another problem caused by the head-forward posture is a misaligned jaw. When the head slips forward, the muscles of the front of the neck pull down on the jaw, causing it to misalign and resulting in a **temporomandibular joint (TMJ)** that does not fit properly. Symptoms of this TMJ misalignment include jaw and throat pain, earaches, and clicking noises when the mouth opens and closes. If someone already has TMJ pain, the

19

head-forward posture will aggravate it further. Thankfully, TMJ pain can be relieved by realigning the head over the shoulders, setting the jaw back into its proper alignment, and relaxing the neck muscles that are pulling the jaw out of place. See Chapter 16 for stretching exercises to relax the neck muscles.

Still more negative consequences of the head-forward posture are disc degeneration and arthritis. When the head is forward of its normal position, the facet joints at the back of the neck will be stretched apart, become inflamed and gradually arthritic. The weight of the head, no longer being carried by the bones of the neck, is transferred to the ligaments and discs. Over time, this will lead to permanent disc damage.

THE CAUSES OF A HEAD-FORWARD POSTURE

Now that you understand the consequences of the head-forward posture, let us examine its most common causes.

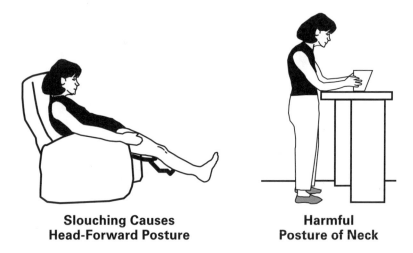

**Slouching Causes
Head-Forward Posture**

**Harmful
Posture of Neck**

A slouched lower back automatically forces your neck to go in the same direction. If you sit in a comfortable chair with your back rounded, your neck will also round and your head will slip forward.

Standing occupations that require a bent-forward, round-shouldered position, such as assembly-line work, hairdressing, and dentistry, often produce a head-forward posture.

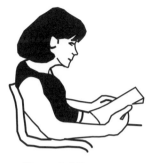

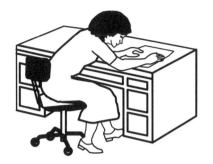

**Harmful Posture
While Reading**

**Prolonged Bending
Over Desk**

Constantly hanging your head forward while reading will result in a head-forward posture. Your muscles will eventually tire and your head will slip forward.

If your occupation requires you to bend over a desk or bench all day, you will eventually develop a head-forward posture.

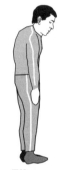

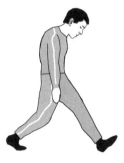

**Elbows
in Front of Midline**

**Looking Down
at the Ground**

If, when you stand or walk, your elbows lie in front of the midline of your trunk, you have a round-shouldered posture. In this posture, the weight of your arms pulls down on your shoulders and upper back, causing your upper back to round. When your upper back is rounded, your head will slide forward. Consider that each arm weighs the same as your head, about twelve pounds. When your head is forward and your shoulders are rounded, your neck is being pulled forward and downward by about thirty-six pounds of body weight!

Sometimes people look at the ground as they walk, instead of looking straight ahead as they should. In this posture, the neck sags, the neck muscles fatigue, muscles and ligaments over-stretch, and the head slips forward.

Wearing high heels pitches the legs forward and thrusts the buttocks backward. To compensate for this architectural realignment, the chest, neck, and head tilt forward. This causes the trapezius muscle to strain to hold the head in place. If this strain continues, the trapezius muscle will become exhausted and the head will slip forward.

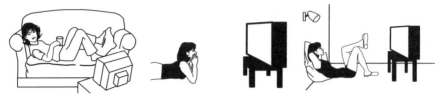

Straining Neck When Lying on Couch   **Straining Neck While Watching TV**

Repetitively watching TV with your head propped up on the headrest of a couch or bed will force your head forward. Lying down to watch TV with your head propped up on your hands or arms will cause the same neck strain. Bending your neck forward repetitively to watch TV also causes neck strain and a head-forward posture.

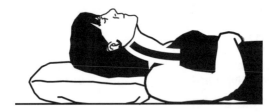

Sleeping on Too-Thick Pillows Causes Neck Strain

It is very common for people with a head-forward posture to sleep with their heads propped up on an extra large pillow or on two or more pillows. While this sleeping posture seems to support their head, it actually puts a continuous forward strain on the muscles of the neck and upper back for the eight hours or so of sleep time, thus worsening the head-forward

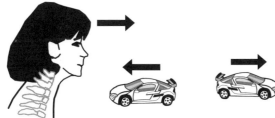
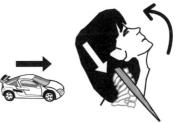

**Head-Forward Posture
Caused by
Automobile Accident**

**Whiplash Neck Strain
Caused by
Automobile Accident**

posture. Once the head-forward posture is corrected by a chiropractor, the thickness or the number of pillows should be reduced.

Automobile accidents often cause a head-forward posture. Front-end accidents fling the skull forward; rear-end accidents pull on the muscles of the front of the lower neck, which attach to the back of the skull. As the head whips backward, these muscles pull the back portion of the skull downward, which forces the front of the skull forward and upward into the head-forward posture.

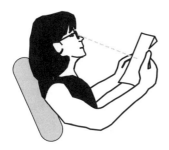
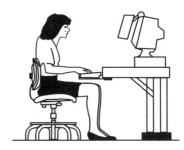

**Backward Bending of Head
Caused by Bifocals**

**Computer Screen Placement
Too Far Away**

People who wear bifocals very often have a head-forward posture, because whenever they focus their eyes on something, they have to lift their head and chin upward to look into the bottom half of their glasses. When they do so repeatedly, they pull their head forward.

Using a computer screen that is too far away from you requires you to repetitively push your head forward and lift your chin up to view the screen.

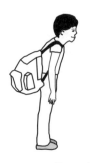

**Improper Carrying
of Backpack**

Sitting at a computer station in which the computer monitor is placed too low will also cause a head-forward posture. See Chapter 14 for more information on proper computer equipment placement.

Children carrying a backpack that is too heavy for their underdeveloped body have to bend over excessively to balance the contents of their bag. When they do so, they push their chin forward, misaligning their posture into the head-forward position.

Normal Posture

CORRECT STANDING POSTURE WHEN OBSERVED FROM THE FRONT

You know you have correct standing posture when:

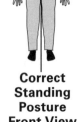

- Your eyes and ears are parallel to (level with) the floor.

- Your head and neck are straight, without leaning to either side.

- Your shoulders and hips are parallel to the floor.

- The bridge of your nose (directly between your eyes), the center of your chin, the notch between your collar bones, the middle of your breast bone, your belly button, the middle of your pubic bones, and the midpoint between your feet are all in a straight vertical line.

**Correct
Standing
Posture
Front View**

CORRECT STANDING POSTURE WHEN OBSERVED FROM THE SIDE

You know you are maintaining correct standing posture, with all four curves of your spine in place, when:

- You are standing straight without bending your neck.

- You are facing straight forward with your eyes looking straight ahead.

- The object you are looking at is clearly visible by looking straight ahead or by simply tilting your eyes up or down.

- Your head is directly above your shoulders.

- Your shoulders are resting comfortably on top of your rib cage.

- Your arms are hanging straight down.

- Your lower back is arched slightly forward.

- Your ear hole, mid shoulder, mid hip, knee, and ankle are in a straight vertical line.

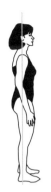

Correct Standing Posture Side View

CORRECT SITTING POSTURE

Correct sitting posture differs at work, at home, and in your vehicle. These various postures will be discussed in Chapters 12, 13, and 14. However, in general, the following apply to correct sitting posture:

- You are sitting up straight, or leaning slightly backward, without bending your neck.

- You are facing straight forward with your eyes straight ahead.

- Your head is directly above your shoulders.

- Your shoulders are resting comfortably on top of your rib cage, not leaning forward or backward.

- Your upper arms are hanging straight down.

- Your lower arms are bent at right angles to your upper arm, parallel to the floor, or with your wrists slightly higher than your elbow joint and supported on the armrests.

- You are sitting all the way back in your chair with your buttocks against the back of the chair, not in the middle or on the front edge.

- Your lower back is slightly arched forward and supported by the back of the chair.

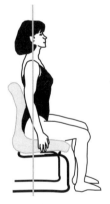

Correct Sitting Posture Side View

- Your knees are slightly higher than your hip joints
- The back of your lower thighs should be one inch above the front edge of the chair seat.
- Your feet are flat on the floor.
- Your ear hole, mid shoulder, and mid hip are in a straight vertical line, or in a line that leans slightly backward at the top.

CORRECT POSTURE WHEN LYING ON YOUR BACK

The normal, healthy posture for lying on your back is the same as the normal standing posture as seen from the side, but lying down.

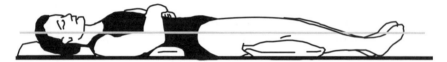

Correct Lying on Back Posture - Side View

- Your face is upward.
- Your lower back and neck are slightly arched.
- Your ear hole, mid shoulder, mid hip, and ankles are in a straight horizontal line.

CORRECT POSTURE WHEN LYING ON YOUR SIDE

The normal posture when lying on your side is almost the same as the normal standing posture as seen from the front, only lying down.

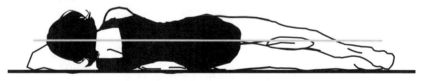

Correct Lying Posture - Back View

- You are looking straight ahead.
- Your neck is parallel to the mattress, not leaning upward or downward.

- The bridge of your nose (directly between your eyes), the center of your chin, the notch between your collar bones, the middle of your breast bone, your belly button, and the middle of your pubic bones are all in a straight horizontal line. This line then slants downwards between your feet.

Tests for Determining Posture
Checking Your Posture from the Front

THE MIRROR TEST

To check your neck posture from the front, do the mirror test. Stand facing a full-length mirror. Place your heels approximately six inches apart. Raise each foot four or five times as if walking in place, stopping in a natural upright stance. (Do not look at your feet.) Close your eyes, move your head forward and backward, then from left to right, stopping in a comfortable position that feels centered. You may now open your eyes, but do not move your head or body. First, observe your ears, nose, and chin to determine whether your head is slightly rotated or facing directly into the mirror. Next, check to see if your head is tilting to one side. You know your head is tilting when your neck is in a straight vertical line yet your eyes or ears are not parallel to the floor. Then, observe your neck in relationship to your upper body. Is your neck leaning to one side with

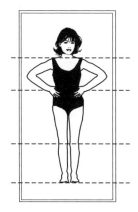

**Mirror Test Revealing
Normal Posture**

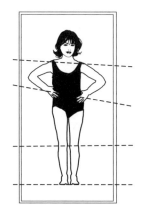

**Mirror Test Revealing
Abnormal Posture**

one eye lower on the side of the lean? Have your head and neck translated (shifted) to one side? In this case, your eyes and shoulders will be parallel with the floor; however, your head and neck have shifted to the side of the centerline of your body. Lastly, look at your shoulders and your hips. They should be level with each other and parallel to the floor. If your head is rotated or tilted, if your neck leans to one side, or if your shoulders or hips are not level, you have posture problems.

Continue the mirror test by checking the relationship of your torso to your pelvis. First, observe if your shoulders and upper body have shifted to one side, with your shoulders and belt line parallel to the floor. If so, the posture of your thorax has slipped into a lateral translation (sideways) position. Next, check to see if your upper body is leaning to one side (lateral flexion). If so, your upper body will be leaning to one side, with one shoulder lower on the side that is leaning and your head will be off-center to the side of the low shoulder. Lastly, determine if your body is rotated. In this case, one shoulder will be closer to the mirror than the other. Once again, if any of these imbalances exist, you have a postural problem.

Checking Your Posture from the Side

THE WALL TEST

This test is a great indicator of good or bad posture from the side. Stand with your back about one foot from a wall. Walk backward slowly until your buttocks, mid back, or head touches the wall. If all three of these do

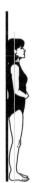

**Wall Test Revealing
Normal Posture - Side View**

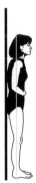

**Wall Test Revealing
Abnormal Posture - Side View**

not touch the wall simultaneously, or if your lower back (at waist level) or mid neck is not one and a half to two inches from the wall, you have a postural problem.

THE SIDE-PICTURE TEST

To do this test, you will need to have someone take a picture of you from the side. Before taking the picture, place a round dot or small piece of paper under your ear hole on the side being photographed. Place a second dot or piece of paper on the middle of the outside of your shoulder joint on the same side, and a third dot or piece of paper on the middle of the top of your leg bone where it attaches to your hip.

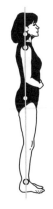

Side Picture Test Revealing Normal Posture

If your posture is good, you will notice in the picture that the dot under your ear hole is directly over the dot on your shoulder. If the dot on the ear is forward of the dot on the shoulder, you have a head-forward posture. If the dot on your ear is further back than the dot on your shoulder, you have a posterior translation (head-backward) posture.

Next, check the posture of your mid back from the side. First, observe whether your entire upper body, as a unit (head, shoulders, and mid back) is forward or backward of your hips. In this case, the dot under your ear hole is directly over the dot on your mid shoulder, yet both of these dots are forward or backward of the dot on your hip joint. This abnormal posture is called anterior (forward) or posterior (backward) translation. Then, check to see if your head and thorax (mid back) are leaning forward or backward in relationship to your pelvis. If the dot under your ear is forward of the dot on your shoulder and both of these dots are forward of the dot on your hip joint, you have an abnormal flexion (forward-bending) posture. If the dot under your ear is behind the dot on your shoulder and both of these dots are behind the dot on your hip joint, you have an extension (backward-bending) posture. Lastly, check to determine if you have a kyphotic (rounded) mid back.

Posture X-Ray Views

These are specific x-ray views taken by a chiropractor who specializes in postural correction. These views determine whether your posture has deviated from normal. This method provides a very accurate determination of any postural problems.

COMPUTER POSTURE-ANALYSIS TEST

Many chiropractors specializing in postural correction have a computer program that analyzes a patient's posture. These doctors take front-view and side-view pictures of you, enter them into their computer, discuss the results with you, and get you on a program to improve any postural problems.

The Neck-Shoulder-Back Connection

In order to change the position of your neck, most of the time you have to change the position and mobility of your shoulders, mid back, and lower back because they are interconnected. Without a forward curve in your lower back, it is almost impossible to have an ideal curve in your neck. A head-forward posture is almost always accompanied by tight shoulders and a slumped, rounded mid back. To properly fix one area, you have to fix the other areas at the same time.

Maintaining Correct Posture

The following instructions will help you maintain correct posture and prevent neck pain.

- Stand up straight with your eyes and chin level when you walk. The goal is to keep your head level rather than looking up or down. Imagine you are trying to touch the sky with the top of your head. Another great technique is to visualize yourself balancing a book on top of your head.

- Place your shoulders directly on top of your rib cage. Imagine a helium balloon attached to the top of your head and one attached to each shoulder. These balloons elongate your neck to make you taller and lift your shoulders. As your head lifts, your neck relaxes, and your shoulders fall into place. Do not push your shoulders forward or backward, just place them on top of your rib cage. Try to hold yourself in this position at all times.

- Avoid locking your knees when you stand. A locked position pushes your hips, lower back, neck, and head forward. Stand with your legs loose or bent slightly, which allows your head and neck to remain in their normal position.

- Neck-proof your environment; in other words, modify your household, work surfaces, and furniture to match your height and build. Neck-proofing will help keep you from bending your neck and body into awkward positions to fit these items. See Chapters 12 through 15 for neck-proofing instructions.

Section Two:

Reducing Neck Strains in Daily Life

3

Using Your Head to Protect Your Neck

As you know by now from reading this book, most neck pain is caused by misalignment of vertebrae or by sore muscles. Many of the daily activities and postures that cause these two problems are directly under your control. In other words, by improving the way you sit, stand, and work, you can greatly reduce your chances of suffering neck pain. With this book, you will become neck-smart. You will learn how to avoid the strains to your neck muscles that could lead to injury. Your journey to an injury-free neck begins by learning two basic neck-care facts.

FACT #1: Repeatedly bending or turning your neck strains it.
To prevent straining your neck in daily life, your work and play surfaces must be at the proper heights to keep you from frequently bending and turning your neck. In addition, the objects you frequently look at need to be in your direct field of vision, so that you are not forced to repeatedly bend or turn your neck to see them. Much of this book deals with modifying your different environments to fit your body.

FACT #2: Overstretching your neck, arm, or shoulder muscles will pull on your neck vertebrae, possibly pulling them out of alignment and causing a neck injury.

In order to prevent your neck, arm, or shoulder muscles from pulling excessively on your neck, the objects you need to grasp or lift should be within your easy reach. Repeated over-stretching can strain your neck muscles.

Positions That Strain Your Neck

PROLONGED POSITIONS

Staying in the same position for an extended period of time will result in muscle tightness, reduced circulation in your muscles, and ultimately muscle pain. If you must hold one position for a length of time, take a break once an hour and perform range-of-motion exercises of your cervical spine. See Chapter 16 for appropriate exercises.

STANDING

Standing for a long period of time, especially on hard floors such as concrete or terrazzo, exhausts the muscles that support your lower back. When these muscles tire, your lower back sags forward into an excessive curve, which then automatically forces your neck into the same excessively curved position. The following tips will reduce the stress on your neck. If you must stand for long periods of time:

→ take breaks

→ transfer your body weight from one foot to the other

→ do mild back-stretching exercises described in Chapter 16

→ stand with one foot on a step stool or foot rail, alternating feet from time to time

PROLONGED LEANING

Leaning your neck to the side for long periods of time causes several problems. It jams your neck bones and pinches the nerves on the side that your neck is leaning toward. It also strains the neck muscles on the side opposite the lean.

A good illustration of this habit is when you cradle a phone between your shoulder and neck rather than holding the phone with your hand or using a headset. The sustained bending of your neck to the side and the raising of your shoulder to hold the phone in place strains your neck muscles and

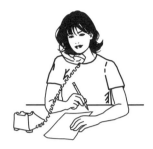

Cradling Telephone Causes Neck Strain

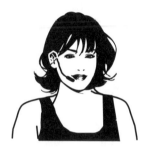

Hands-Free Headset

pinches the nerves that go into your arms, hands, and fingers, potentially resulting in a numbness and tingling of your arms and fingers. This position also strains your upper back and shoulder muscles, producing pain and misaligning your spinal vertebrae.

To avoid neck and upper back strain when talking on the telephone, follow these neck-care tips: Place the arm that is holding the telephone on its elbow on a surface that is high enough to hold the telephone receiver at your ear level while keeping your neck in the normal upright position, or hold the telephone to your ear while your neck is in the normal posture, switching sides as necessary to avoid muscle strain. These actions will help keep your neck aligned. Or, if you regularly talk on the telephone for long durations, use a hands-free headset[508] or a speakerphone[501]. These devices eliminate the need for cradling the phone and free your hands, allowing your neck to always stay in an aligned position.

Leaning your chin on your hands while sitting at a desk or table is another bad habit that you should become conscious of breaking. This position not only strains your neck but also may allow your jaw or vertebrae to slip out of alignment. If your neck is tired, take a break and do some of the neck-stretching exercises described in Chapter 16.

PROLONGED TURNING

Very little rotation occurs naturally in your neck except for in the top two vertebrae. Turning your head for long periods of time stretches and weakens the muscles, ligaments, and joints of your neck. Examples may include when talking with someone sitting to one side of you, rotating your neck to face an individual, turning your head to face a pastor speaking to a congregation or a teacher lecturing to a classroom, or turning your head to use a computer monitor that is placed at your side. This extended position strains your neck and forces your vertebrae to slip out of alignment.

Instead of twisting your neck when you need to see something or someone not in your direct field of vision, turn your body as a unit and face the object or person with your whole body. This is summed up in a simple rule: Your nose and toes should always point at an object you are looking at or lifting.

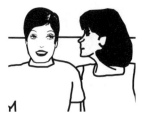

Prolonged Rotation Causes Neck Strain

PROLONGED FORWARD BENDING

Repetitively bending your head forward can be a difficult habit to break. Most activities involve leaning the head forward, or forward and down, for example, writing, reading, knitting, sewing, sitting on the floor to work or play, and playing games. The problem is that prolonged forward bending compresses the discs of your neck, places an unnecessary strain on your neck and upper back muscles, and forces your neck ligaments to hold up the weight of your head and neck—a

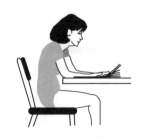

Avoid Prolonged Forward Bending of Neck

job they are not designed to do. As a general guideline to prevent neck damage and pain, avoid bending your head forward for more than thirty seconds at a time. Another helpful tip is to bring the object you are viewing up to eye level as much as possible.

WATCHING TV

Poor posture while watching TV or reading places more stress on your neck than almost any other activity. Hanging your head forward for ex-

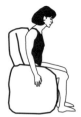

Television Placed Too Low Causes Neck Strain

tended periods of time to watch TV while seated, or lying down on a couch with your head propped up on the armrest, or lying in bed with your head propped up on multiple pillows or the headboard, will force the normal forward curve of your neck to become reversed. These postures bend your neck too much, stretching the muscles and

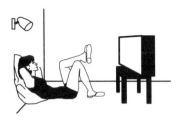

**Straining Neck
While Watching TV**

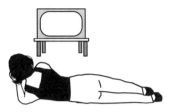

**Propping Head on Hands
Causes Neck Strain**

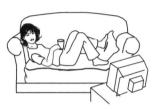

**Head on Arm of Couch
Causes Neck Strain**

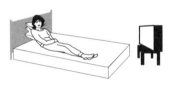

**Head on Headboard
Causes Neck Strain**

ligaments of your neck and producing a strain on your neck muscles.

Never lie on your stomach with your head propped up in your hands or lie on your side to watch TV with your head propped up on your hand and arm. These positions will strain your neck as well as kink your neck backward or to one side. The nerves on the kinked side will be pinched. The muscles on the other side will be stretched. Both positions will eventually produce pain. To eliminate these injuries, break the habit of lying down to watch TV. Also, sitting on the floor and looking up or sitting in a chair looking down at a TV tilts your head too much. Place your TV in a position so that your head is neither tilting up nor down. By not tilting your neck up and down, you help prevent neck problems.

READING

Many people who read a great deal experience neck pain as well as pain in the upper back or between the shoulder blades. No other activity places your neck in a prolonged and motionless stressful posture as much as reading does. Reading postures can create havoc on your neck and mid back muscles.

The best practice is sitting up to read with your reading material placed directly in front of you at slightly below eye level. A slantboard [503] may also

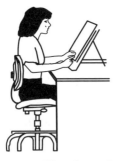

Use a Slantboard

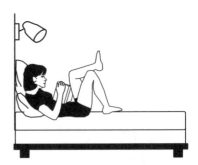

**Propping Head on Headboard
Causes Neck Strain**

be used to help prevent bending your neck forward to see the page. Resting your elbows on a desk while you read also relaxes your neck muscles.

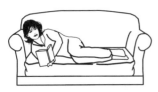

**Head on Armrest
Causes Neck Strain**

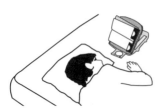

**Side Reading
Slantboard**

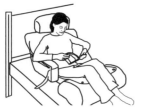

Body Support Lounger

On the other hand, reading in bed with your head propped against the headboard bends your neck forward too far. This sharp angle will strain your muscles and misalign your neck vertebrae if held for extended periods.

Lying on your side to read with your head propped up on an armrest of a couch or on your hand has the same effect as lying on your stomach with your chin and head propped up on your hands; these positions severely stretch your neck muscles and ligaments, misalign vertebrae, pinch nerves, and produce neck pain. For those who like to read in this position, there are special side-reading slantboards[400] that allow you to lie on your side to read while keeping your spine in correct alignment.

If you insist on reading or watching TV in bed, use a special body support bed lounger[401]. This device helps keep your spine correctly aligned. Place your reading material up on a reading pillow[402] rather than

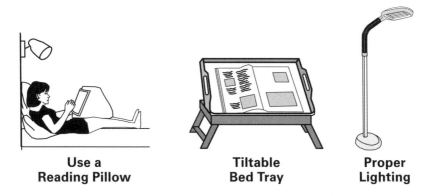

**Use a
Reading Pillow**

**Tiltable
Bed Tray**

**Proper
Lighting**

at lap level. By doing this, you avoid bending your head and neck too far forward and downward. Placing your reading material on a tiltable bed tray [403] also helps keep your neck straight and in alignment. It is also beneficial to place your elbows on a pillow to relax your trapezius muscle (the muscle that goes from the back of your head to your shoulders).

Proper lighting is essential for stress-free reading. When reading while sitting in a chair, use lighting that simulates the balanced spectrums of natural daylight [404]. When reading in bed, use a book light [405] attached directly to your book. Reading with poor lighting forces your face closer to the pages of the book, placing a strain on your neck.

PROLONGED BACKWARD BENDING

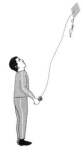

**Prolonged
Backward
Bending of
Neck Causes
Neck Strain**

Bending your neck backward for long periods of time, such as when looking directly overhead, puts a tremendous strain on the muscles and ligaments at the front of your neck, compresses the discs and facets at the back of your neck, and pinches the nerves that go out of your neck into your shoulders, arms, and hands. Always try to avoid bending your neck backward for more than thirty seconds at a time.

Activities that cause excessive backward bending of your neck include drinking from bottles, cans, or narrow-mouthed glasses (instead, drink from a wide-mouth container or use a straw); shaving; brushing

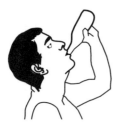

**Drinking from
Bottle Causes
Neck Strain**

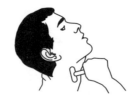

**Neck Strain
Caused by Shaving**

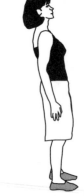

**Correct Method of
Looking Upward**

your teeth; applying makeup; propping your chin on your hands; or reaching overhead.

If you need to look upward for extended periods of time, lean your entire body backward by pushing your stomach forward and keeping your head and neck relatively straight.

SITTING

The main guideline to follow when sitting is to sit up straight, look straight ahead, and keep the curves of your spine in their normal position. Slumping or slouching is one of the worst things you can do to your neck.

If you must stay seated for long periods of time, change your position as frequently as possible. Better yet—if you do not have to remain seated— stand up, walk around for a few minutes, or do range-of-motion exercises

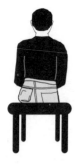

**Sitting on
a Wallet**

(see Chapter 16). When you talk on the telephone, walk around as much as you can. You do not have to be seated to talk on the telephone or to have a conversation with somebody.

Do not let objects get in your way of maintaining a healthy posture. For example, sitting with a large bill-fold in your back pocket will raise your pelvis higher on one side every time you sit. Over time, this will cause your lower back to shift in one direction and your neck to shift in the opposite direction, straining and possibly misaligning it.

Movements That Strain Your Neck

Your next challenge is to modify your lifestyle and establish new **"neck-wise"** habits to prevent future neck-attacks.

REPETITIOUS MOVEMENTS

Repetitious movements are a common source of neck strain. Repeated lifting, pushing, pulling, digging, sweeping, bending, or twisting will abnormally pull and stretch your muscles. If you must do the same movement over and over again, alternate the side of your body that is doing the work. For example, alternate your hands on the handle of a shovel, broom, or vacuum cleaner and alternate your feet when digging. Do what you can to equalize the burden placed on your neck, shoulders, and arms.

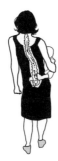 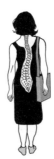

Harmful Posture While Carrying Baby **Incorrect Placement of Shoulder Strap**

The same guideline applies to any repetitive activity that places stress on only one side of the body, such as carrying a baby on one hip or wearing the strap of a purse over one shoulder. Give each side of the body equal time so that you avoid stressing one side too much.

WALKING

Rather than stomping, "glide" or "float" as you walk. The lighter you walk, the less noise your feet make and the less you will jar your spine (producing less micro-trauma), and the less the walking action will hurt your neck. Avoid bouncing because it, too, produces micro-trauma that can hurt the discs and vertebrae of your neck.

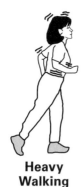

Heavy Walking Produces Micro-Trauma

Bending your knees as you walk acts as a shock absorber for your spine. Conversely, locking your knees tends to jar your body. It also forces your lower back to bend excessively forward, thus forcing your neck into the same unhealthy posture. Always try to keep your knees slightly bent as you walk or stand.

To further prevent micro-trauma to your neck, wear soft-soled shoes and, when possible, stay on carpeted areas and limit the amount of walking you do on hard surfaces, particularly concrete, pavement, tile, or terrazzo floors.

Jogging also produces micro-trauma and can aggravate the tissues of your neck.

STOOPING

Avoid stooping when you have a neck problem. Whenever you stoop, your neck and head hang on your neck ligaments and muscles, stretching the ligaments and straining the muscles.

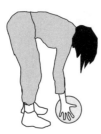

Don't Stoop

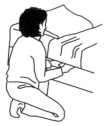

Squat to Make Bed

A safer technique for bending downward is to squat. Squat whenever you have to pick up objects off the floor, make beds, do laundry, get into low cupboards, or do gardening work. Squat when looking into low file cabinets or reaching into low drawers and shelves at work. Squatting allows your neck and back curves to be maintained, which will significantly reduce the chance of injury.

In order to squat safely, you must always face the object. Place one foot slightly in front of the other, shoulder-width apart. Maintain your spinal curves with your back and shoulders straight. If you can, give yourself extra support and balance by placing a chair next to you or resting your hand on a table or countertop. This will ease the strain to your muscles while squatting.

44

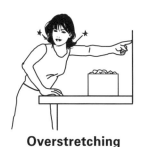

**Overstretching
Causes
Neck Strain**

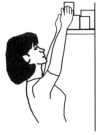

**Avoid
Reaching Above
Shoulder Level**

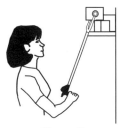

**Use of
"Reaching Stick"**

REACHING AND STRETCHING

Any activity that requires reaching or stretching more than twenty inches places a great strain and tension on the muscles and ligaments of your neck. To avoid this, move frequently used objects within close reach or move closer to the objects before reaching for them.

Avoid reaching for anything that is above your shoulder level, for example, trying to remove something from a high shelf. Whenever you reach above your head, you throw your head and neck backward, stressing your neck muscles and compressing the facets at the back of your neck. Change this habit by keeping your arms at shoulder level or below. When you have to reach for something above shoulder height, stand on a ladder or step stool[406] and face the object to be reached. Use a long-handled reaching stick[407] to reach items that you cannot easily grasp.

Working with your arms above your head, such as when nailing or painting, can also place a tremendous strain on your neck. In this scenario, stand as close to your work area as possible. You should also take brief, frequent breaks from this position to avoid excessive strain and fatigue.

When reaching for something that is behind you, remember to turn your entire body to face the object before reaching for it. This method will eliminate unnecessary stress on your neck, arms, and shoulders.

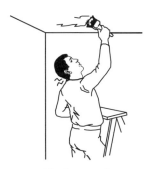

**Prolonged
Looking Upward
Causes Neck Strain**

TURNING OR TWISTING YOUR HEAD AND NECK

As discussed, you should avoid turning your neck for prolonged periods of time. To keep your neck healthy, you also need to be conscientious about not twisting your neck quickly or beyond its normal limits. Twisting your neck beyond its normal limits stretches and strains the joints of your neck, strains your neck muscles, and produces shearing stress on the discs and facets of your neck. To avoid injury, turn your neck within your pain-free range of motion.

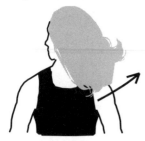

Don't Whip Hair Over Shoulder

People with long hair have a tendency of whipping their head to one side to throw their hair over their shoulder, which can overstretch their neck muscles and ligaments, injure their facets, and possibly misalign their neck vertebrae. A safer technique is to grasp and move the hair with their hands.

Another important neck rule is to not twist your neck when reaching for something—for example, when reaching into a drawer, picking something up from off a table, or pulling up weeds. As always, if you want something that is at your side, turn your entire body to face the object and then grasp it.

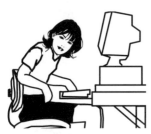

Avoid Bending, Twisting, and Leaning of Neck

One of the worst things you can do to your neck is to bend, lean, and twist all at the same time. When done together, as when looking over your shoulder at something on the ground behind you, these coupled movements place significant rotational and shearing force on the muscles, facet joints, and discs. Sprains and vertebral misalignments are more likely to occur when you are bending, lifting, and twisting simultaneously.

SUDDEN MOVEMENTS

Finally, seemingly simple actions or sudden movements, such as flopping into a chair, sofa, or bed, can injure your neck. Avoid these types of movements altogether to ensure a healthy, pain-free neck.

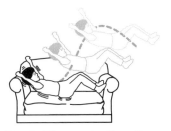

Don't Flop onto Furniture

Another sudden motion that frequently injures the neck is sneezing. If your neck is turned, or not consciously tightened when you sneeze, you will likely strain your neck muscles and discs. When sneezing, follow these rules: straighten your neck, face straight ahead (make sure your nose and toes are facing in the same direction), tighten your neck muscles … then sneeze.

The neck-aids and neck-appliances described in this chapter can be ordered through your family chiropractor or from the Neck and Back Products store at **www.NeckAndBackProducts.com** or call toll-free **1-800-882-4476**.

4

Reducing Neck Strains
While Sleeping

In Section One, we looked at how crucial proper posture is for preventing neck and back pain. Correct posture keeps the muscles and ligaments of the neck and spine healthy and the vertebrae in alignment. Similarly, maintaining proper posture while sleeping is equally important, especially when you consider that, on average, we spend about one-third of our lives sleeping—that is about twenty-five years! There is no getting around it: to maintain a healthy body, you need to have correct postural support while sleeping.

Because this book is about preventing neck pain, my first and foremost concern about sleeping with poor posture is that it places stress on the sensitive soft tissues of the neck and strains the neck muscles. Additional negative effects include numbness and tingling down the arms as well as headaches.

Fortunately, there are many neck-appliances and neck-aids available on the market to correct the posture of your spine during sleep.

So, what can you do to maintain correct posture during the eight or so hours you sleep each night? The first step is to use a pillow that will adequately support your neck while you sleep. When your head is comfortably cradled in the ideal support position by a pillow of the proper type, size, and shape, your neck muscles will not need to stretch abnormally and thus will not be strained.

Other special pillows support the curve of the lower back and reduce the pull of the knees that occurs in various sleeping positions. These types of supports are also important to a healthy neck because if your lower back is allowed to sag into an abnormal position while sleeping, stress will also be placed on your neck. Often these additional pillows are needed to maintain proper sleeping posture.

If you cannot sleep because your neck hurts, it usually indicates that your neck is not being properly supported during sleep. This is a warning sign that your sleep posture is straining your neck muscles, that one or more of your neck vertebrae are out of alignment, or that some other problem needs to be corrected. Simply put, correct sleeping posture relaxes your neck muscles; incorrect sleeping posture strains your neck muscles and causes pain.

Correct Posture for Common Sleeping Positions

SLEEPING ON YOUR BACK

Characteristics of an ideal posture while sleeping on your back, as discussed in Chapter 2, are:

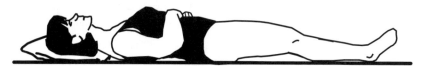

Correct Back-Sleeping Posture

- Your face is toward the ceiling.
- Your lower back and neck are slightly arched.
- Your ear hole, mid shoulder, mid hip, and ankles are in a straight horizontal line.

The best posture while lying on your back is achieved using several aids, including a proper-sized contour pillow [408] under your neck (or a combination of a thin pillow under your head with a cervical roll [409] under your

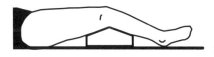

"Knee-elevator" Pillow

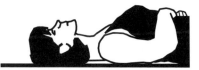

**Avoid Sleeping
Without a Pillow**

neck), a small pillow or a "Night Roll" [410] under your lower back, and a "knee elevator pillow" [411] under your knees.

Sleeping on your back without a pillow under your neck, with a pillow that is too thin, or without the proper-sized pillow/cervical roll combination will cause your neck to sag toward the mattress, flattening the natural curve of your neck and straining your neck muscles.

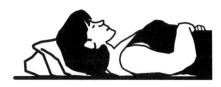

**Sleeping on Multiple Pillows
Causes Neck Strain**

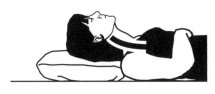

**Sleeping on Too-Thick Pillows
Causes Neck Strain**

Using a pillow that is too thick or using more than one pillow under your head and neck when you are in the back-lying position will push your head up and bend your neck forward. This position strains your neck muscles and stresses the facets at the back of your neck. Many commonly used pillows are too thick, especially for sleeping on the back.

If you sleep on your back, most of the support of a contour pillow or pillow/cervical roll combination should be under your neck, not your head. Additionally, putting a pillow under your shoulders will push your neck into a backward-bending position, aggravating it. Putting a pillow only under your head with no support for your neck will bend your neck forward, straining it. Always place your pillow under both your neck and head, with the majority of the support being under your neck.

The pillows that support your neck and head need to be the thickness that is correct for *your* body. If you sleep on your back, you can

51

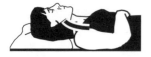

**Pillow Placed
Too High**

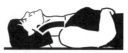

**Pillow Under
Shoulders Causes
Neck Strain**

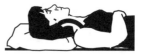

**Correct Placement
of Pillow**

determine the correct thickness of a pillow by performing another "Wall Test." Stand with your back against a wall and measure the distance between your neck (not your head) and the wall. A properly support-

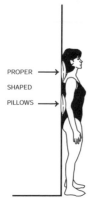

PROPER ⟶
SHAPED
PILLOWS ⟶

**Wall Test
Revealing
Pillow Sizes**

ive pillow when compressed should be thick enough to fill this space. If you choose a contour pillow, one in which the edges of the pillow are thicker than the center, the edge of the pillow should be thick enough, when compressed, to fill the space between your neck and the wall. The center of the pillow should be thick enough, when compressed, to fill the space between your head and the wall.

Because it is so important to maintain the curves of the spine and neck, it is unwise to sleep on your back without a pillow under your neck. A "Night Roll" un-der your lower back and a "knee elevator" pillow under your knees would be even more beneficial. Without the support of a "Night Roll," your lower back will gradually flatten out against your bed. When this hap-

pens, your neck will also flatten, becoming strained in the process. When your knees are slightly bent from the support of a "knee elevator" pillow, the strain on your lower back and neck will be largely relieved.

Another bad habit that occurs while sleeping on your back is sleeping with one or both of your arms behind or above your head. These positions

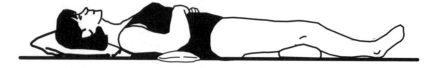

Use of Pillows for Back-Sleeping

prop up your head and bend your neck forward, causing a strain on your neck muscles, compressing your neck vertebrae, and stretching your neck ligaments. Your arm, or arms, will ultimately "go to sleep" due to nerve impingement. If you awaken in the morning with pain or numbness in your arms, this indicates that you were sleeping too long with your arms above your head or that

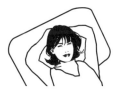

Don't Sleep with Arms Overhead

you have a pinched nerve in your lower neck. A pinched nerve can lead to more serious problems. If the sensation recurs, check with your chiropractor immediately to determine its cause. A good trick to train yourself not to place your arms behind or above your head is to pin the sleeves of your pajamas to the sides of your pajamas.

SLEEPING ON YOUR STOMACH

Never sleep on your stomach. This position twists your neck all night, sprains your neck, pulls your neck vertebrae out of place, compresses the discs and nerves of your neck, and may contribute to certain types of headaches. This posture can also compress the blood vessels of your neck. Sleeping on your stomach is a significant contributing factor to neurological or vascular problems and produces an accumulating strain.

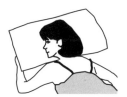

Stomach Sleeping Causes Neck Strain

If you are in the habit of sleeping on your stomach, break the habit by sleeping with a large "positioning wedge" [412]. Another trick is to sew large buttons in the shape of large balls on the front of your pajamas. When you attempt to roll onto your stomach, the buttons and "positioning wedge" will stop you.

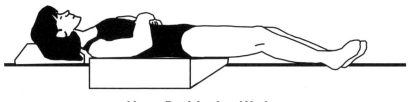

Use a Positioning Wedge

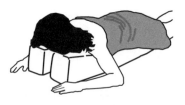

Stomach-Sleeping Pillow

Sometimes it takes time to train yourself not to sleep on your stomach. If you consciously know you are not supposed to sleep on your stomach, eventually it will become "automatic" to roll onto your back or side.

If you cannot break the stomach sleeping habit, sleep on a special stomach sleeping pillow[413]. This special pillow allows you to sleep facedown while still being able to breathe normally. These stomach sleeping pillows also insure proper postural support because you do not have to turn your neck while sleeping.

SLEEPING ON YOUR SIDE

Characteristics of an ideal posture while sleeping on your side, as discussed in Chapter 2, are:

- You are looking straight ahead.

- Your neck is parallel to the mattress, not leaning upward or downward.

- The bridge of your nose (directly between your eyes), the center of your chin, the notch between your collar bones, the middle of your breast bone, your belly button, and the middle of your pubic bones are all in a straight horizontal line. This line then drops from your mid pelvis to a midpoint between your feet.

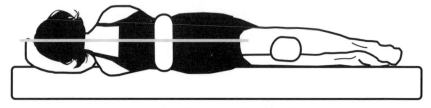

Analyzing Side-Sleeping Posture from Back

The side-lying posture is an excellent position for sleeping, as long as the proper-sized pillow or pillow/roll combination props up your head and neck to become level with your mid and lower spine. Sometimes, special waist and knee pillows are needed to attain the ideal side-lying sleeping posture. It is also a good idea to bend your knees forty-five degrees when lying on your side, as this position will relax your back muscles.

Never sleep on your side without a pillow under your head and neck. Doing so forces your neck to bend toward the bed and subsequently strains your neck muscles. If you sleep on your side, you need a thick pillow to fill the wide gap between your neck and the mattress. This will keep your spine properly aligned throughout the night.

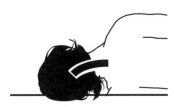

Sleeping Without a Pillow Causes Neck Strain

To determine the proper thickness of your pillow for sleeping on your side, lie on one side in front of a mirror and visualize a straight horizontal line between the middle of your forehead, the notch of your breastbone (between your collar bones), and the centerline of your chest. If this imaginary line is tilted too far upward at your head, your pillow is too thick. If this line is tilted too far downward at your head, your pillow is too thin.

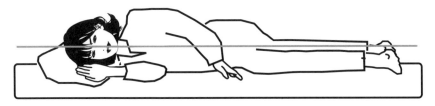

Analyzing Side-Sleeping Posture from Front

Another way to find a pillow of the best thickness for sleeping on your side is to have another person stand behind you and observe how your head and neck line up with your body while you try pillows of different heights. The other person will be able to determine the proper-size pillow to raise the midpoint of the back of your head to the height where your neck attaches to your body.

Never sleep on your side with your arm under your head or pillow or with your elbow above your ear. This will strain your neck and shoulder muscles. If you find that you are sleeping in this position, it is a sign that

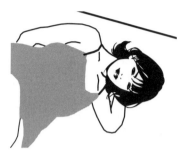

Don't Sleep with Hands Under Head

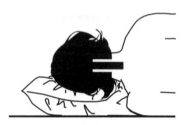

Correct Thickness of Pillow

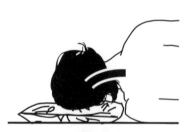

Too-Thin Pillow Causes Neck Strain

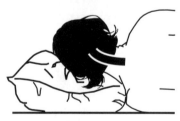

Too-Thick Pillow Causes Neck Strain

you are not getting the support you need from your pillow and that you need a thicker pillow.

CHOOSING A PILLOW THAT IS RIGHT FOR YOU

Neck pain that starts when you are sleeping is primarily caused by the leaning of your neck toward the bed or by your neck hanging unsupported (sagging). This sagging and leaning pinches the nerves and strains the muscles of your neck, producing pain. You can eliminate the sagging, leaning, or straining by using the correct pillows. Likewise, sleeping on your side with your head supported too far upward will also strain your neck.

The most important thing to remember when choosing a pillow is that you want to support the natural curves of your neck and spine and keep your vertebrae in alignment while you sleep. By knowing your body type and what kinds of pillows are available, you can select pillows that will work best for you.

TYPES OF CERVICAL PILLOWS

Because people come in different shapes and sizes, one type of pillow could never meet everyone's posture-support needs. Different types of cervical pillows made from various materials are used to comfortably cradle the head and maintain the neck in its neutral, healthy position throughout the night. The following is a comprehensive list of available neck pillows.

Foam-Rubber Pillows

Sleeping on a foam-rubber pillow that is flat (not contoured to support the neck) will raise your head too high. This kind of pillow is also too firm; it pushes back against the weight of your head and neck. In response, your head and neck will push against the pillow, trying to get into a comfortable position. This back-and-forth pressure causes a strain on your neck muscles, exhausting them. Sleeping on one of these foam pillows results in an eight-hour strain on your neck. Simply using one can be a major source of neck pain.

If you insist on using a foam-rubber pillow, you will need to replace it every six months; the foam compresses and the pillow becomes too thin, thus not giving your head and neck proper support.

Down, Kapok, or Feather Pillows

Many doctors prescribe down, kapok [414], or feather pillows because these types of stuffing are very pliable. By pushing in the center of the pillow, you can make a hollow mold for your head to fit into. The rest of the material will bunch up around the edge to support your neck. However, avoid loosely filled or thin pillows because there will not be enough down, kapok, or feathers to bunch up under your neck, leaving your neck unsupported. Down or feather pillows called "Sneeze-Inducers" are not recommended for people who have allergies.

Cervical Contour Pillows

Cervical contour pillows [408] are designed to properly support your head and neck while you sleep on your back as well as when you sleep on your side. Cervical contour pillows provide excellent support and thus prevent you from straining your neck while sleeping.

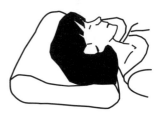

Contour Pillow

Cervical contour pillows are made of special foam rubber or "memory foam." These pillows have an indentation in the middle for the head and raised edges around the indentation to support the curve of the neck. This design allows the neck muscles to relax and the neck to rest in alignment with the rest of the spine. If you tend to change positions during the night, a cervical contour pillow is an excellent choice for you.

If you have difficulty getting used to a cervical contour pillow, talk with your chiropractor. The inability to sleep with your head and neck properly supported is a warning sign that a vertebra in your neck is out of alignment or that your muscles are strained. Do not allow any discomfort to go unanswered. Ultimately, if any pillow continues to hurt your neck, discontinue its use and seek chiropractic care.

Pillow/Cervical Roll Combination

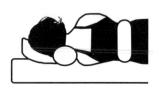

Cervical Roll/Pillow Combination

Some doctors prefer to prescribe a cervical roll [409] instead of a cervical contour pillow. When you lie on your back, place the roll behind your neck with your head resting on a thin pillow. Similarly, when you sleep on your side, again place the roll under your neck with your head resting on the thin pillow. This can be easily accomplished by tucking a "neck roll" into the pillowcase of a flat, soft pillow. This combination of a cervical roll and thin pillow beneath your neck and head, respectively, should hold them in proper alignment with the rest of your spine.

Be sure that your cervical roll is of the correct thickness when compressed. The correct thickness will provide almost total relief from neck strain. The size of the roll will depend on how much space there is to be filled. If either the cervical roll or pillow is too thick, your neck will arch upward, creating a stress on your neck. If this occurs, reduce the size of both pillows. The most common mistake is using a roll that is too small. If the combination of thin pillow and roll allows your neck to sag, the pillow and roll need to be thicker. On average, the correct size of a cervical roll is about five to six inches thick and sixteen inches wide.

The cervical roll should be soft to allow your neck to sink into it. One that is too hard or too large will push your neck upward, straining it.

Visco-Elastic (Memory-Foam) Pillows

High-density visco elastic (memory foam) is five times denser than ordinary foam. A high-density visco-elastic pillow [415] uses your own body heat to mold itself gently to the curves of your neck and head within five to ten minutes. The pillow supports your spine in normal posture while eliminating pressure points on your head and neck. This is important because pressure points can interfere with sleep. This benefit has made this type of pillow the standard in many chiropractors' offices, sleep centers, and hospitals in the United States and Europe.

Water Pillows

Water pillows [416] provide responsive head and neck support. The weight of the head indents the middle of the pillow, pushing the water to the edges of the pillow. The edges then get thicker and, as a result, better support the neck. A water pillow will automatically conform to your changing sleeping positions

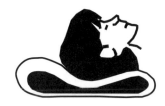

Water Pillow

throughout the night. The thickness can be controlled by the amount of water inserted into the thin water bag in the middle of the pillow. A thick polyester fiber covering rests over the water layer.

One necessary precaution when using a water pillow is that it is heavier than a feather, foam, or air pillow, and the weight can be a hazard if you try to move the pillow during the night by pushing it with your head, as this may strain your neck muscles. However, if you move the pillow with your hands, you will not have a problem.

Air Pillows

You can add air to these types of pillows by squeezing a bulb. You control the thickness of the pillow by the amount of air you pump into it. An air pillow supports your neck correctly, reduces pressure points, and helps maintain blood flow to your muscles.

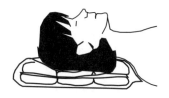

Air Pillow with Multiple Bladders

Air pillows come in two types. The first is similar to a typical contour pillow—with raised edges and an indented center. Air can be pumped in to thicken the edges and center [417]. The second type of air pillow has multiple air bladders within the pillow [418]. Not only can the pumped-in air control the thickness and firmness of the pillow, but also these bladders automatically adjust to the pressure of your head, just like a water pillow does. The weight of your head pushes down on the air bladders in the middle of the pillow, forcing some of the air out of the central air bladders into the air bladders that make up the rim of the pillow, which support your neck.

The air pillow may be your pillow of choice if you travel frequently. You can deflate the pillow for easy packing and pump it up when you reach your destination, thus insuring proper neck support during sleep.

SIDE-SLEEPING PILLOWS

Special side-sleeping pillows [419] have been designed to properly support the neck when sleeping on your side. These pillows have shoulder cradles that maximize cervical support, facial relief pockets, and special air channels that make breathing easier.

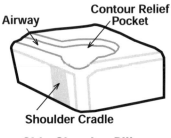

Side-Sleeping Pillow

Travel Pillows [420]

Special pillows that support your neck while traveling in a vehicle or airplane are described in Chapter 10.

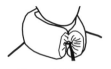

Travel Pillow

PILLOW FIRMNESS

A pillow that is too soft will compress too much, allowing your neck to sag toward the mattress, straining it. A pillow that is too hard or too thick will force your head in the opposite direction, again, straining your neck.

If you sleep primarily on your back, you will need a soft pillow that allows your head to push into it. If you are primarily a side sleeper, you will need a firm pillow to fill the gap between your neck and the mattress.

LIFE EXPECTANCY OF PILLOWS

Unfortunately, pillows do not last a person's lifetime. High-quality pillows can last five to ten years. Inexpensive pillows will last only a few nights to six months. When your pillow no longer gives you the support you need, change it.

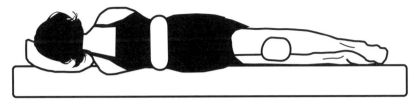

Cervical, Waist, and Knee Pillows

BODY TYPES
Wide Shoulders

If you sleep on your side and have wide shoulders, you will need a thicker contour pillow, side-sleeping pillow, or pillow/cervical roll combination to raise your head and neck into proper alignment. If you have a narrow waistline and wide shoulders (an hourglass figure), you may also need a small "Night Roll" at your waistline to properly raise your lower spine to the level of your upper spine when sleeping on your side. Remember, if your lower spine sags, so will your neck. With an hourglass figure, you may also need to use a contoured knee pillow [421] between your knees. When your knees and upper legs sag downward, they pull on your pelvis and lower spine. The lower spine becomes stressed, which automatically stresses your neck.

Narrow Shoulders

If you sleep on your side and have narrow shoulders, you will need a thinner contour pillow, side-sleeping pillow, or pillow/cervical roll combination to properly support your head and neck.

Head-Forward Posture

As discussed, healthy standing posture, when analyzed from the side, is when the ear hole is directly over the mid shoulder. Chronically poor posture, accidents, and injuries sometimes force our heads to shift forward. People who have a head-forward posture will need to use more than one pillow, a thicker contour pillow, or a thicker pillow/cervical roll combination when sleeping on their back until their head-forward posture is corrected.

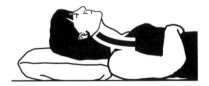

Sleeping on Too-Thick Pillows Causes Neck Strain

This thicker pillow should be thick enough to support the head, but not too thick. A pillow that is too thick will push the head more forward, aggravating or worsening the head-forward posture.

If you have a head-forward posture, it is best to sleep on your side to reduce the stress on your neck.

Mattresses

As noted, we spend approximately one-third of our lives in bed. Therefore, it is crucial to the health of your neck and spine to choose the right mattress. The key is to always sleep on a relatively "hard" mattress that will not sag in the middle. A sagging mattress permits your lower back to sag, and, as you know by now, when your lower back sags your entire spine is affected, including your neck. However, be careful that a mattress is not overly firm. A mattress that is too firm will flatten the curves of your neck and back, producing pain and stiffness. The ideal mattress is one that is firm and has a pad affixed to its top.

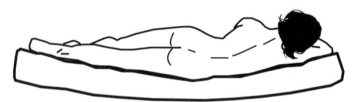

Too-Soft Bed Causes Poor Sleeping Posture

MATTRESS TYPES

Water beds, visco-elastic (memory-foam) mattresses, multiple density foam (multi-zone) mattresses, inner-spring mattresses, and airbeds can adequately support your back and neck. The following are mattresses that chiropractors recommend, as they provide excellent support.

Visco-Elastic (Memory-Foam) Mattresses

As noted in the discussion on pillows, high-density visco elastic (memory foam) is five times denser than ordinary foam. Like the pillows, a high-density visco-elastic mattress [422] uses your own body heat to mold itself gently to your curves within five to ten minutes, giving support to your spine in normal posture while eliminating pressure points on your body. As mentioned, this is important because pressure points can interfere with sleep. The memory-foam mattress is the standard in many sleep centers and hospitals in the United States and Europe.

Multi-Zone Mattresses and Springs

The multi-zone mattress and springs [423] combines the features of the visco-elastic mattress with three to five different densities of high-density latex foam. The highest-density foam is used to support the hip and lower back area, providing extra-firm back support. The mid back area, being lighter, has a medium density foam. And, because the head and leg areas require less support, they are supported by a lower-density latex foam.

Inner-Spring Mattresses and Springs

In general, inner-spring mattresses and springs [424] provide excellent support for the spine. However, these beds offer various degrees of support—the number of springs within the mattress determines the amount of back support you receive. The average bed has only 900 springs—which provides adequate support for only a short time. This is because the weight of your body gradually compresses the springs until the support becomes inadequate. For longer-lasting and better support, we recommend mattresses that have a greater number of springs.

Air Mattresses

An air mattress [425] has easy-to-use hand controls that pump air into an airbag until it reaches the desired firmness. Air mattresses conform to your every curve, giving you excellent postural support and thus reducing the pressure points that can create a restless sleep.

Air mattresses give couples an extra advantage: each side of a King- or Queen-size airbed can be adjusted to the comfort level of the person sleeping on that side. If you use an air mattress, make sure it is not pumped too firm. Recommended is an air mattress that has a thick, soft "cushion" stitched to the top of the sleeping surface.

Water Beds

Water beds [426] can also provide excellent support for your back and neck. However, the less expensive the bed, the less support it usually gives.

When using a water bed, make sure you pump enough water into the bed to make it the firmness you need. An under-filled water bed will allow your spine to sag, injuring your spinal tissues. Better-quality water beds have baffles in them to prevent the wave action that occurs when someone gets in and out of the bed or turns over. This wave action can strain your neck muscles. Some water beds have baffles on both sides of the mattress, allowing the firmness on each side to be controlled separately.

If you are considering getting a water bed, make sure the sides of the bed are firm; otherwise, you may stress your neck muscles getting out of it. Also, make sure the bed has a heater to control the water temperature. Cold water will cause your neck and back muscles to tense—and tense muscles, over a period of time, ache.

MATTRESS RULES

If your bed is sagging, it is time to throw it away. Most mattresses need to be replaced every five to eight years, no matter how good their warranties are. Inexpensive mattresses will wear out even more quickly.

Never place a board between your mattress and the box springs. This will make your bed too firm. Instead of conforming to your spine, a mattress that is too firm will "iron out" your spine's natural curves.

A King-size mattress is always the ideal, so that your sleeping partner will not jar you during the night.

Couch and Chair Sleeping

As comfortable as it may feel, lying down on a couch with your head on the armrest is a habit that is important to break. The armrest is too high for you to maintain good posture; your head gets pushed forward, and your neck muscles become stretched and strained.

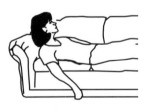

**Don't Lie with
Head on Armrest**

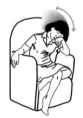

**Don't Sleep
in Sitting Position**

If you fall asleep sitting up in a chair, your head will "bob" up and down or fall forward or to one side, again, straining your neck muscles and possibly causing your vertebrae to move out of alignment.

One way to safely sleep sitting up in a chair is to support your neck properly using a travel pillow [420] or crescent-shaped pillow [427]. These

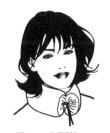

Travel Pillow

pillow-like aids will prevent your neck from bobbing up and down, falling forward or to one side, and, therefore, will allow you to sleep in a seated position without injuring your neck.

Neck Rules for Sleeping

In addition to using the proper pillows and mattress, following these important guidelines will contribute greatly to a lifetime free of neck pain:

- Get in and out of bed properly. Some people flop into bed, jarring their neck. Instead, sit on the edge of the bed and gently lower yourself down.

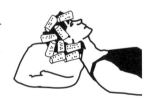

Don't Flop into Bed

- Never roll over in bed by pushing up on your head and using it as a pivot. Rather, roll over by raising your head off the pillow and then turning your shoulders, trunk, and head as one unit.

- When you get out of bed, turn onto your side and use your hands to push yourself upward into the sitting position. This helps you avoid using your neck muscles.

- When your neck hurts, avoid sleeping in one position for an extended period of time. Change your sleeping positions from one side position to the other or from a side position to a back position, and so on. This will increase the blood supply to your muscles and avoid further neck strain.

Sleeping on Curlers Causes Neck Strain

- Avoid sleeping with large curlers in your hair; they will prop your head up too high, straining your neck muscles. Curlers are also uncomfortable and will force you to twist and turn all night, interfering with your rest.

- No matter what position you sleep in, use only one pillow under your head. More than one pillow will force your head too high and overstretch your neck tissues. As noted, the exception to this rule is when an individual has a head-forward posture.

The neck-aids and neck-appliances described in this chapter can be ordered through your family chiropractor or from the Neck and Back Products store at **www.NeckAndBackProducts.com** or call toll-free **1-800-882-4476.**

5

Household Activities
That Can Strain Your Neck

Without knowing it, you may be causing the onset of neck problems and pain by the way you are performing your everyday activities.

Many common household activities can strain your neck muscles. By merely changing only slightly how you do these activities you can greatly reduce the chances of hurting your neck. Although a little tedious at first, adopting these new, healthy ways of performing daily activities is ultimately being very "neck-smart." Your neck will thank you!

House Cleaning Activities

VACUUMING, SWEEPING, AND MOPPING

Vacuuming, sweeping, and mopping have the potential to over-stretch your neck muscles, straining them. During these activities, you bend, lean, and twist at the same time. As you know from information covered so far, this combination of motions can be very stressful to the joints of your neck.

Vacuuming

When you vacuum, follow these basic posture guidelines: Stand up as straight as you can and keep your neck aligned with the rest of your

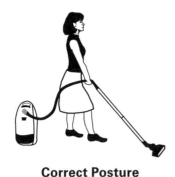

**Correct Posture
While Vacuuming**

body. Bend forward at the hips, but not too far forward, and bend your knees slightly. Keep your head upward, and step forward with the vacuum, the same way fencers step forward when they lunge, using the leg on the same side as the hand you are using to hold the vacuum.

Vacuum in a straight, forward-and-back motion with minimal side-to-side movement. If you use a canister-type vacuum, hold the wand—the long, thin tube between the end of the cleaning hose and the carpet brush—close to your hips to prevent straining your neck. Avoid twisting to one side, and alternate the hand and the side of the body doing all the work. Try not to lean over the vacuum, because you will be hanging your head and neck on your ligaments and straining your muscles. Ideally, if you use a canister vacuum, make sure it has a wand long enough that you can vacuum standing up straight. Using a long-handled wand also allows you to move your arm, rather than twisting your neck and body, to vacuum around objects.

Another important key to safe vacuuming is to limit the distance you vacuum to one foot at a time. The further you reach, the more you will strain your neck. Additionally, yanking on the hose to reposition the vacuum can hurt your neck muscles. Instead, walk back to the vacuum cleaner and reposition it when necessary.

If your vacuum of choice is an upright model, choose a self-propelled one. Self-propelled vacuums automatically move themselves forward or backward with just a slight touch of the handle. This greatly reduces the amount of muscle you will need to use and thereby reduces your risk of straining your neck.

Better yet, use a self-propelled, robotic vacuum cleaner. This machine automatically moves around the floor, cleaning as it goes with virtually no human effort required. With a robotic vacuum cleaner, you will not strain your neck because the machine does all the work—you do no pulling or pushing. Buy a robotic vacuum cleaner [428] and let it do the work for you.

One last tip about vacuuming: If your house is more than one story, either have a central vacuum system installed or store a separate vacuum cleaner on each level so that you do not have to lift or carry a heavy vacuum up and down the stairs as you vacuum from floor to floor.

Sweeping and Mopping

A good way to avoid over-stretching your neck muscles when sweeping and mopping is to use an ergonomically correct push broom[429], a combination broom and motorized dustpan[430], or mop[431] instead of a regular broom or mop. These special push brooms and mops are easier to use and eliminate the excessive twisting that can injure your neck.

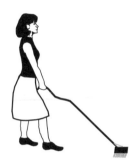

Use an Ergonomic Push Broom

When sweeping or mopping, stand erect, keep your head up, hold the broom or mop close to your body, and alternate the side of the body doing all the work. And, as with vacuuming, limit the distance you cover to one foot at a time.

Or, use a self-propelled, robotic floor-washing machine. This machine automatically moves around the floor, scrubbing and cleaning with virtually no human effort required. With a robotic floor-washing machine, you will not strain your neck because the machine does all of the work—you do no pulling or pushing. You can buy a robotic floor washer[432] and have your floors washed with no effort on your part!

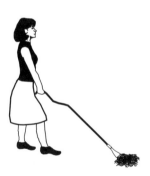

Use an Ergonomic Mop

DOING LAUNDRY

Pulling wet clothes out of a washer may strain your neck. When you do laundry, do several small loads instead of one large, heavy load. Then, empty your washing machine in stages—wet clothes are heavy and the pulling and lifting of anything heavy can create havoc on your neck. The smaller and lighter the load, the less pulling and straining you will have to do.

Always bend your knees and hip joints when pulling heavy laundry out of the washing machine. Whenever you bend your knees and hip joints, you reduce the strain on your lower back, which also reduces the strain on your neck.

IRONING

When you iron clothes for a long period of time, the weight of the iron in your hand can pull on your neck, straining your neck muscles. In addition, you will probably have your head leaning downward while ironing, which increases the stress on your neck. Another good tip is to take extra steps when ironing a long item, such as the sleeve of a tall man's shirt, instead of stretching your arm out to the end of the sleeve. Overstretching while holding a heavy iron places considerable stress on your neck muscles. In addition, consider breaking up your ironing into smaller batches to avoid spending too much time at once on this task and thereby overstressing your neck muscles.

MAKING THE BED

The key to safely making a bed is to avoid bending your head and neck forward many times or reaching too far across the bed. Bending creates neck discomfort because, to accomplish this posture, your head and neck are hanging on your ligaments, stressing them. Reaching too far, of course, may overstretch the muscles of your back and neck. If your bed is against a wall, pull it at least one and a half feet away from the wall so you can go around to the other side easily rather than having to reach all the way across the bed to make it.

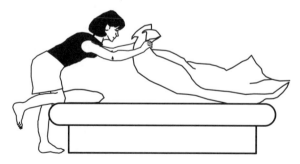

Correct Method of Making Bed

To make your bed without straining your neck, place one knee on the bed and bend downward by pushing backward with your buttocks while keeping your back straight. By assuming this posture, you will be able to accomplish your task more comfortably without placing stress on your neck. When straightening the covers or adjusting the pillows on your bed, do one side at a time. Pulling too hard on your sheets, blankets, and covers, and bending and twisting to tuck in the sheets, can also strain your neck muscles. Take your time and get as close as possible to the object you are pulling to keep your neck muscles safe.

Lawn Maintenance

MOWING THE LAWN

The most neck-friendly way to mow your lawn is to use a self-propelled lawn mower that has a starter switch. This will allow you to avoid jerking a cord to start the mower, thus better protecting your neck. Most of the neck strain produced by a mower occurs by using one that has to be pushed and pulled.

It is least desirable for you to mow your lawn using a riding lawnmower. Even if

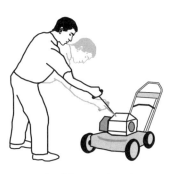

**Jerking a Cord
to Start a Lawnmower**

your model boasts great shock absorption, it will still create an excessive amount of vibration that can lead to painful disc degeneration in your neck and back.

WEEDING

To avoid neck strain caused by weeding, use a long-handled weeder instead of bending your neck forward and downward when pulling out the weeds by hand. Kneeling on the ground or bending at the waist for long periods can cause muscle strain and lead to injury.

RAKING AND HOEING

Raking and hoeing require constant use of your neck and shoulder muscles, and thus can be very stressful to your neck. To minimize the stress caused by raking or hoeing, follow these guidelines:

- Keep your knees slightly bent.

- Place your feet one foot apart.

- Position one foot ahead of the other.

- Frequently alternate which foot is in front.

- Squat downward slightly with your back straight. This position will allow you to use your thigh muscles more and decreases the stress on your neck and back.

- Use a lightweight, ergonomically designed, long-handled garden rake [433] or hoe [434] with a two-hand grasp attachment for easier handling. The shafts on these tools are bent at angles that allow for a stronger grasp, which produces less strain on your neck.

- Keep the rake or hoe and your arms close to your body.

- Move the rake or hoe forward and backward, shifting your weight from one foot to the other; use your feet more and your back less.

Use of Ergonomic Rake

- Alternate the rake or hoe and your hand placement from one side of your body to the other.

- Do not reach too far in front of you with the rake or hoe.

- Drag the leaves to you.

- Do not twist your body.

- If your raking job is a big one, use a leaf blower.

- For big hoeing jobs, use a gasoline-powered hoe (Rotatiller) to assist you.

GARDENING

When most people do gardening, they stoop down with their head and neck bent forward to reach the plants and flowers on the ground. Bending forward for extended periods of time, of course, strains your neck quite a bit. To avoid bending your head and neck forward and downward while gardening, plant your vegetables and flowers in elevated lightweight plastic planters, elevated flowerpots, or window boxes.

If you still prefer to garden the old-fashioned way—kneeling on the ground—invest in a portable garden seat [435] or a rolling garden seat [436]. These devices enable you to sit closer to the ground, thereby reducing your need to bend and thus the strain to your neck.

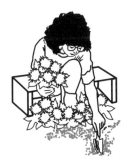

Garden Seat

When gardening, it is especially important to remember some of the general posture and neck-care guidelines we have covered in the book so far:

- Face every task with your whole body. Keep your nose and feet pointed toward the objects you are gardening.

- Keep your head and neck in the neutral position, because twisting and flexing your neck as you pull weeds can strain your neck.

- Keep your knees and hips slightly bent.

- Reduce the amount you have to bend at the waist and minimize bending your head and neck forward.

- Never lift and twist simultaneously.

- Do not sit on the ground with your back rounded and your head hanging forward on its ligaments; instead, kneel on one knee and put one hand on the ground for support.

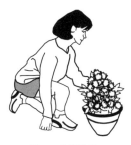

Kneel While Gardening

SHOVELING AND DIGGING

Shovel and dig in soil cautiously. Pulling on a shovel and twisting to throw dirt can easily strain your neck.

Follow these shoveling guidelines to avoid hurting your neck:

- Rather than shoveling hard-packed soil, loosen it first with the shovel or simply add some water to the soil. Fresh, moistened, or loose soil (moistened soil *is* loose) is the easiest to shovel. While it is wise to moisten the soil first to make it softer, do not add so much water that the soil turns to mud. Mud is heavy and is much harder on your neck to shovel than is loose soil.

- Make sure your shovel is as sharp as a knife.

- Use an ergonomically correct shovel [437] with a handle on it. The shaft on this tool is bent at an angle that allows for a stronger grasp, which produces less strain on your neck.

- Place one hand mid-shaft for easier shoveling.

- Shovel only small amounts. Large amounts are too heavy and can strain your neck muscles.

- Do not reach or stretch. Move closer to the area where you are digging.

- Keep the loaded shovel as close to your body as possible.

- Bend at your knees and hips, keeping your back and neck straight.

- Use your thigh as a fulcrum (teeter-totter) for tougher digging.

- Do not twist your neck while lifting the contents of the shovel.

- Alternate your hands and feet frequently to avoid excessive strain on one side of your body.

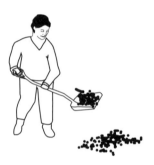

Proper Use of Shovel

- Only throw the soil you are shoveling a short distance from your body. The further you throw the soil, the more you will strain your neck muscles.

- Take frequent breaks to rest your muscles.

USING A WHEELBARROW

If you are using a wheelbarrow to carry dirt or plants, keep your loads light; lifting a heavy load can strain your neck muscles. A wheelbarrow with large wheels [438] reduces strain on

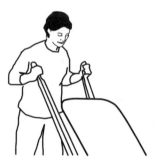

Proper Way to Empty Wheelbarrow

your neck and back. Making more trips with smaller loads is less convenient; however, a pain-free neck is well worth the extra effort. When you dump the contents of your wheelbarrow, dump the load straight ahead and keep your body facing forward rather than twisting it to the side.

USING A GARDEN HOSE

To eliminate stress on your neck caused by yanking, pulling, and rewinding lawn hoses, get an automatic rewinding garden hose device [439]. These devices rewind your hoses with the flip of a switch. An alternative to an automatically rewinding garden hose is a coiled hose [440]. These hoses take up less space and are easier to manage than uncoiled hoses.

TRIMMING SHRUBS, BUSHES, AND TREES

Regular hand trimmers place considerable strain on your neck muscles. To eliminate this strain, use a power trimmer to trim your shrubs and bushes. The newest trimmers and pruners have soft-grip handles that are shaped to fit your hands, producing less stress on your arms and neck. To avoid looking overhead when trimming trees, stand on a ladder or scaffold and use a power trimmer with a long handle.

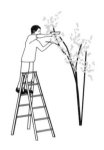

Stand on Ladder to Trim Trees

House Maintenance Activities

WATERING PLANTS

Neck-smart plant-watering tips are easy to implement. First, put only a small amount of water in the watering can at a time. Carrying and holding a full watering can will cause similar stress on your neck as holding a heavy iron. Next, stand up straight when you water your plants. Use a watering can that has a long spout to avoid leaning over your plants to water them. Finally, arrange your plants so you do not have to bend your head and neck forward to water them.

USING TOOLS

When possible, use cordless tools. Pulling and yanking electric cords can strain your neck muscles.

Store all tools at a height that you can reach by simply extending your arms forward. Therefore, you will not have to bend your head and neck forward to grasp your tools. Better yet, store your tools in a lightweight, rolling tool organizer or carrier [441]. Using rolling carriers eliminates the need to lift tools, such as rakes, hoes, and shovels, thus reducing unnecessary stress on your neck.

REMOVING SNOW

For those of you living in a climate that receives snow, you know what a chore shoveling this heavy stuff can be—and what a strain it can place on your neck and back muscles. One way to make removing snow easier on your body is to use a push blade with wheels [442], a snow scoop [443], or a push snow shovel [444] instead of a typical snow shovel. Shoveling strains your neck muscles, but pushing does not. If the snow is too deep, use a snow blower to clear your path.

Follow these snow-shoveling guidelines to avoid hurting your neck:

- Try to shovel the snow when there is only a little snow on the ground, no more than two to four inches. It will be looser and lighter. You will, of course, have to shovel more often during a snowstorm, but this is healthier for your neck and back than is lifting heavy snow.

**Use a
Push Snow Shovel**

- Never shovel hard-packed, partially frozen snow. Only shovel loose snow. Hard-packed snow, or frozen snow, is too heavy. Breaking it loose, then lifting a heavily loaded shovel will hurt your neck muscles.

- Push the snow to the side of a walkway or driveway, rather than shoveling the snow.

- Make sure your shovel is as sharp as a knife.

- Use an ergonomically correct shovel [437] with a handle on it.

- Place one hand mid-shaft for easier shoveling.

- Shovel only small amounts. Large amounts are too heavy and can strain your neck muscles.

- Do not reach or stretch. Move closer to the area you are shoveling.

- Keep the loaded shovel as close to your body as possible.

- Bend at the knees and hips, keeping your back and neck straight.

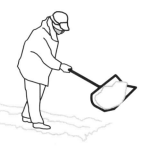

**Only Throw Snow
a Short Distance**

- Use your thigh as a fulcrum (teeter-totter) for tougher shoveling.

- Do not twist your neck while lifting the contents of the shovel.

- Alternate your hands and feet frequently.

- Only throw the snow you are shoveling a short distance from your body. The further you throw the snow, the more you will strain your neck muscles.

- Take frequent breaks to rest your muscles.

PAINTING/NAILING

As you have learned, looking upward jams the facets of your neck together and may irritate your spinal nerves. When having to do overhead work, it is always wise to use a ladder or scaffolding. Move the ladder or scaffolding often in order to keep your body as close to your work as possible. Long-handled tools also help with these tasks. Painting or nailing anything overhead forces your lower back to bend backward, which causes you to bend your neck forward, straining it. Overhead work can invite neck problems, especially if you have to reach,

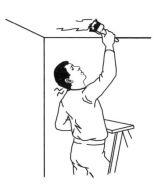

**Prolonged Looking
Upward Causes
Neck Strain**

twist, or put your body in an awkward position. Prolonged periods in this position will place excessive stress on your ligaments and muscles.

Pet Care

When you walk your dog, use a leash that stretches. This will reduce the sharp jarring of your neck that can occur with a regular leash.

Kitchen Activities

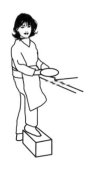

**Use Step Stool
When Doing Dishes**

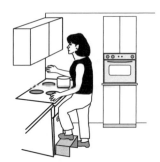

**Use Step Stool
While Cooking**

COOKING

When you cook or wash dishes, rest one foot on a low step stool [406] or on the edge of an open drawer. This will place your back and neck in the properly aligned position.

As a general rule, if anything has to be lifted or moved in the kitchen, follow these four steps: 1) Face the object, 2) keep your neck and back straight, 3) pull the object close to your body, and 4) lift the object with the strength of your arms and legs.

If possible, avoid using heavy cookware. If your cookware is heavy, slide and pull the heavy pots and pans to you before lifting them. This will avoid any unnecessary strain on your neck muscles.

CLEARING THE TABLE

When clearing a large table, it is very easy to over-reach and twist to grasp dishes and other objects from around the table. This usually entails hanging your head downward on the ligaments and muscles of your neck, which, as you

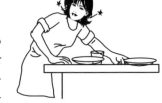

Avoid Over-Stretching

know, can stress the ligaments and strain the muscles. To keep your neck healthy, always clear one side of the table first, then the other side. This way you only have to reach a short distance from your body.

WASHING DISHES

Standing over a sink to wash dishes by hand requires prolonged forward bending of your head and neck, and thus can strain your neck muscles. A better choice for your neck is to use a dishwasher, when possible.

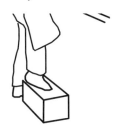

Use Step Stool When Doing Dishes

When placing items into a dishwasher, remember to face the dishwasher when loading it. Do not twist your neck to the side when loading it. If you must wash your dishes by hand, place one foot on a six- to ten-inch step stool[406] or open the cabinet door under your sink and place one foot on the bottom edge of the cabinet. Alternate your feet every few minutes. This technique will help keep your back straight and help prevent your neck from bending forward, thus reducing the strain on your neck.

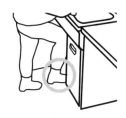

Place Foot on Bottom Edge of Cabinet

TAKING OUT THE TRASH

As you know, the strain of lifting anything can injure your neck. When you take out the trash, bundle your garbage into smaller, more manageable packages. Make several trips with small bundles rather than one trip with a large, bulky bundle.

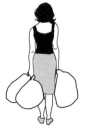

Correct Lifting of Trash Bags

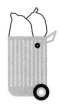

Trash Can on Wheels

Use a trashcan on wheels or a wheelbarrow when transferring trash bags. The lifting and pulling of trash bags can strain your neck muscles.

Sometimes it is too difficult to get the trash out of a compactor. The pulling and jerking used to get a heavy trash bag out of a trash compactor may injure your neck. If you use a trash compactor, do not fill it all the way up. Throw out partial loads.

GROCERY SHOPPING

As with anything you have to carry, bag your groceries in small loads. Heavy grocery bags will pull on your neck muscles. Always push the grocery cart rather than pulling it. Use good posture when pushing the cart—stand up straight and keep your neck straight.

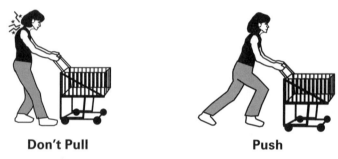

Don't Pull **Push**

If you really want to protect your neck when grocery shopping, shop only at stores that have carts with shallow baskets that are placed higher on the cart. As you know, the more you have to bend over, the more you will strain your neck.

When taking grocery bags out of the cart, place the bags on the rim of the grocery cart as an intermediate step, move closer to the grocery bag, pull it toward you, and then lift. Lifting in this manner will prevent you from bending your neck forward and, therefore, will be easier on your neck.

The neck-aids and neck-appliances described in this chapter can be ordered through your family chiropractor or from the Neck and Back Products store at **www.NeckAndBackProducts.com** or call toll-free **1-800-882-4476.**

6

Personal Care Activities That Can Cause Neck Pain

The number one neck-care rule for personal care activities is to avoid twisting to button or zip clothes, to adjust belts and pants, or to wash yourself in the shower. Next in importance is to avoid repeatedly bending your head forward or holding your head in a bent-forward position for extended periods of time.

Clothing

See Chapter 12 to learn how to properly place your clothes in a closet to prevent aggravating or causing neck pain.

LOOSE CLOTHING

This may sound extreme, but wearing loose-fitting, easily adjustable, and easily donned clothes, such as jogging suits and bulky sweaters, can prevent neck pain. Your twisting and tugging to reach zippers or buttons or pulling on tight clothes may stretch your neck muscles, straining them and producing neck pain.

**Avoid
Awkward Zipping**

WARM CLOTHING

Heat makes muscles relax; cold makes them contract. By keeping your neck and back properly clothed in cold weather, you can avoid painful muscle spasms. If your neck muscles are exposed to very cold weather, they may contract to the point of actually pulling your vertebrae out of alignment.

Shoes

TYPES OF SHOES

Wearing slip-on shoes, such as slippers or loafers, prevents the pulling on your neck muscles that can occur when tying shoelaces. If you wear tie-up shoes, get elastic shoelaces that do not require tying. This makes an ordinary shoe function like a slip-on shoe.

To best protect your neck from the mini-shocks of walking, wear silicone cushions, rubber shoe inserts, soft soles, or add orthotics [702] (special orthopedic appliances that go in your shoes that dramatically reduce the stress of walking, standing, or running). Doctors of chiropractic are trained to evaluate your footwear. If your shoes are old and worn out, every step may be causing micro-trauma to your neck. Your chiropractor can measure your feet and prescribe an orthotic that will be made specifically for you, or you can order custom orthotics from the Neck and Back Products store. If you have to stand or work on hard floors (e.g., cement, tile, terrazzo), you will greatly benefit from wearing soft-soled shoes, which soften the micro-trauma caused by walking. The more micro-trauma your neck experiences, the more the discs of your neck will be damaged.

Avoid wearing high heels or platform shoes, as they force your neck and back into an abnormally forward-bending posture, straining your neck.

PUTTING ON SHOES

To avoid straining your neck when putting on your shoes, place one of your shoes on a chair seat, keeping your head and neck straight up. Then, use a long-handled shoehorn [446] to put your foot into your shoe. Repeat the process to put on your other shoe. Bending your neck and head forward to put on shoes without a shoehorn can strain your neck.

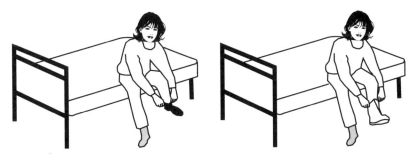

Straining Neck While Putting on Shoes   **Straining Neck While Putting on Boots**

PUTTING ON BOOTS

Be careful when putting on boots; they are hard to get on and off. The effort of pulling on the boots can strain your neck, and because boots often have higher heels than shoes, wearing them will throw your neck and back into an excessively forward position, straining them both.

HATS

If you like to wear hats, make sure to only wear light ones. Heavy hats, if worn long enough, can strain your neck muscles and compress your neck vertebrae and discs. Always tilt the brim of your hat upward so you can see and avoid low objects in your direct path. Tilting your hat also prevents you from having to tilt your head up (and thus bend your neck) to view objects.

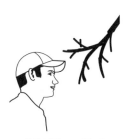

Tilt Your Hat Upward

PURSES AND BRIEFCASES

Ladies beware: Shoulder-strap purses pull on your shoulder and neck, placing a strain on the muscles of these areas. If you do choose to wear a shoulder-strap purse, place the shoulder strap around your neck on the opposite side of your body as the purse, so that the strap falls across your chest. Otherwise, especially if you are round-shouldered, your purse will have a tendency to slip, and you will be constantly hiking your shoulder up to try to keep the strap in place. This motion will cause a constant strain on your shoulder and neck muscles. Better yet, wear

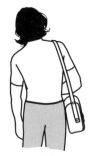 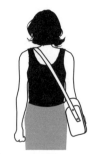 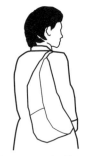

Incorrect Placement   **Correct Placement**   **Ergonomic Purse**
of Shoulder Strap   **of Shoulder Strap**

an ergonomically correct shoulder purse [447]. When you wear this type purse, the weight of it is distributed evenly over the length of the bag's shoulder strap, reducing the load you are carrying on any part of your body by 50 percent.

If you do wear a shoulder-strap purse, make sure it is as light as possible. The straps of heavy shoulder-strap purses will produce pain in your neck by pulling down on your neck muscles. Frequently switching the strap from shoulder to shoulder will minimize the strain put on either side.

Carrying a clutch purse is a better alternative; however, here too, keep it light. Carrying a heavy handbag puts considerable stress on your shoulders, which in turn puts a good deal of strain on your neck muscles and contributes to poor posture—and may even pull your neck out of alignment. Minimize the amount of time you have to carry a heavy handbag and make a habit of keeping your shoulders level while holding on to your purse. Switch your handbag from hand to hand frequently to lessen the strain put on one side.

Also, you can try switching to a fanny pack; they place the weight on your hips instead of your shoulders.

Similarly, avoid overloading a briefcase or suitcase, making it too heavy, because it will pull on one side of your neck, straining it. And, as always, alternate the weight from one hand to the other.

Ergonomically correct briefcases [448] are also available. These reduce the stress on your shoulders by 67 percent. If you must carry your briefcase a considerable distance, I recommend using this type.

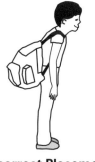

**Incorrect Placement
of Backpack**

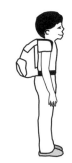

**Ergonomically
Correct Backpack**

BACKPACKS

This goes for men, women, and children: Avoid most backpacks. The majority of backpacks pull your upper back backward, sending your head and neck excessively forward, straining your neck. Instead, use special ergonomically correct backpacks [449] that do not injure your neck or upper back.

Especially harmful is carrying a backpack over one shoulder. This will pull your neck and shoulder downward, straining them. If you want to wear a backpack, wear it properly—over both shoulders.

Women's Clothing

PUTTING ON A BRA

The most neck-friendly way to put on a bra is by hooking the bra in front of you and then turning it around and putting your arms and shoulders through the straps. At the same time, keeping your neck and back straight, lean forward by pushing backward with your buttocks and let your breasts fill the cups. Then stand up, again keeping your neck and back straight. Another option is to wear bras that hook in the front.

Avoid bras with narrow shoulder straps, as they will cause pain in your neck, shoulders, and upper back. If you are big-breasted, get specially made bras or place pads underneath the shoulder straps; otherwise, the shoulder straps will cut into your upper back muscles, forcing you to drop your shoulders

Bra Strap Pads

downward and to round your shoulders to get away from the pain of the straps. This causes your neck to bend forward—and may even cause your skull to slip forward. As explained in Chapter 2, this head-forward position throws your entire posture off and strains your neck muscles. Also, change your posture by stretching your chest muscles and tightening your mid back muscles by following the exercises in Chapter 16.

PANTYHOSE, STOCKINGS, AND SOCKS

The best way to put on pantyhose or stockings is while lying on your back. Be conscientious not to strain your neck muscles while pulling them up.

Similarly, avoid twisting your neck while putting on socks. Never bend your head and neck toward the floor to put on your socks. Rather, when putting on your socks, sit up straight and bring the back of your feet up to your buttocks by placing your heels on the edge of the bed or on a chair. To reach your feet more easily, you can lie on your back and bring your knees into your chest.

SHOES

The ideal shoes have one-inch heels and one-quarter-inch soles. Flat shoes, such as moccasins, cause the curve in your neck to straighten, producing stress to your neck. Shoes with heels higher than one inch, and especially those with spiked heels, alter the alignment of your spine from the ground up, forcing your neck into the head-forward position that stresses your neck muscles. The higher the heel, the greater the strain on your neck.

Men's Clothing

SOCKS

Reduce the wearing of long socks, unless they are prescribed by your doctor. The effort involved in pulling up long socks can strain your neck. As a habit, wear loose, short socks.

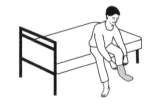

**Pulling on Socks
Can Cause Neck Strain**

SHOES

To further prevent micro-trauma to your neck, wear low-soled shoes and avoid heels higher than one inch. The higher the heel, the greater the strain on your neck and back.

WALLETS

As mentioned, sitting on a wallet that is in your back pocket will elevate one hip, bending your spine to one side while bending your neck in the opposite direction. This will put a strain on your neck and possibly misalign it. The thicker the wallet, the more problems it will cause.

TIGHT COLLARS

Do not wear tight collars, as they can cause a stiff neck as well as tension headaches.

In the Bathroom

The bathroom is a likely place to experience neck strain. You probably spend a lot of time bending over the sink brushing your teeth, washing your face, putting on makeup, shaving, washing your hands, and so on. In a bent-forward position, your head—which weighs ten to fourteen pounds—must be held up by your ligaments and muscles, straining your neck.

VANITIES AND SINKS

An activity such as brushing your teeth or washing your hands places a lot of stress on your neck because most vanities and sinks are built too low and require you to bend forty-five degrees forward. In this case, your neck tissues must bear the entire weight of your head, and the bending-forward position may injure these tissues.

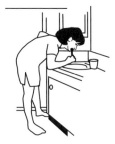

Incorrect Posture When Brushing Teeth

To protect your neck, when you need to bend down to groom yourself, face the sink or vanity, and then bend over by pushing your buttocks backward while keeping your neck and back straight. To return to a standing position, keep your knees bent and bring your buttocks back under you, and you will straighten up without bending your neck. You may also place a hand on the countertop to support your weight and keep your neck in alignment with the rest of your body. This posture will help prevent you from straining your neck.

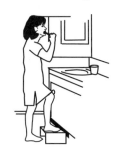

Correct Posture When Brushing Teeth

If you need to stand in front of the mirror or sink for long periods of time, open the vanity or cabinet door and place one foot on the edge of the cabinet, or do the same using a small step stool[406]. This posture maintains the curves of your lower back and neck.

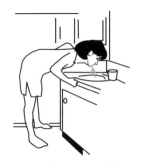

**Correct Posture When
Spitting Out Toothpaste**

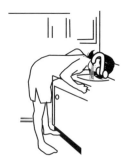

**Drinking from Water Spigot
Causes Neck Strain**

BRUSHING YOUR TEETH

Stand up straight to brush your teeth. When you want to spit out the toothpaste, bend at your knees, push backward with your buttocks, keep your neck straight, and support yourself by placing one hand on the counter—then spit. After rinsing your mouth, return to the standing position by keeping your knees bent and bringing your buttocks back under you.

Never drink out of the faucet to rinse your mouth, as this position places your vertebrae in an extremely awkward, twisted, and bent position, straining your neck muscles and stretching the joints of your neck.

WASHING YOUR FACE

Washing your face by leaning over to splash water from the sink bends your head and neck forward and places a strain on your neck. To wash your face in a neck-friendly manner, stand up straight and use a washcloth.

SHAVING

Avoid bending over the sink to shave. Instead, stand up straight and use an electric razor. Or, shave in the shower with the aid of a fog-free mirror[450]. Try not to tilt your head too far upward when shaving under your chin, as this will strain your neck.

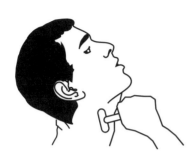

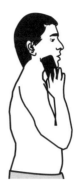

Neck Strain Caused by Shaving   **Use an Electric Razor**

If you have to shave over the sink, get close to the mirror and support yourself with one hand. Then, use a washcloth to rinse your face after shaving.

BATHING
Tub Bath
Lying down to soak or bathe in a tub of hot water for long periods of time will hurt your neck. The curved shape of the tub will force your head and neck into an unnatural, bent-forward position, straining your neck and allowing your vertebrae to slip out of alignment. Take a shower instead.

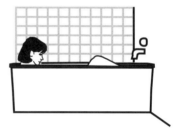

Prolonged Lying in Bathtub Causes Neck Strain

If, however, you do choose to take a bath, do not lie down in the tub. Rather, sit up straight in the tub. If you want to relax, do so in bed, not in the tub.

Most people have difficulty getting out of a tub. Slipping and sliding as you attempt to get out of a wet tub can strain your neck muscles. Therefore, when you get out of a tub, follow these neck-smart safety tips: Empty the tub first. Then, keeping your neck straight, turn over onto your hands and knees and crawl up and out of the tub. Use caution to avoid slipping. Better yet, have a grab-bar installed on the wall near your bathtub for extra support.

Make sure there is a non-skid mat [451] or bottom in your tub. Even if you do not fall, any sudden movement to prevent yourself from falling can strain your neck muscles.

Shower

Your most neck-friendly choice for bathing is to take a shower. Showering, unlike taking a bath, gives you a better opportunity to maintain your normal posture and thus minimizes the stress you place on your neck muscles.

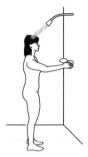

Face the Showerhead

Following are some good showering tips. Use a long-handled scrub brush [452] to prevent twisting as you bathe yourself. Also, when washing your hair, face the showerhead to prevent bending your head backward. If you have to bend forward to shampoo long hair in the shower, do not sling your head backward to get your hair out of your face—this will whiplash your neck. Rinse your hair in the shower by standing up straight with your head and neck in alignment with the rest of your spine.

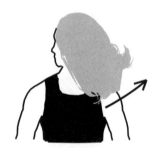

Don't Sling Hair Backward

Make sure you check the water temperature before you enter the shower. Stepping into a shower that is too hot or too cold may force you to suddenly jerk, which can cause a sprain or produce pain if you have an unstable neck.

If you must awkwardly bend your neck and back to stretch for your shampoo, conditioner, etc., have triangular shower shelves [453] installed at shoulder level into the corner of your shower, or purchase shower shelves that affix to your shower-

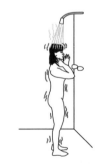

Always Check Water Temperature First

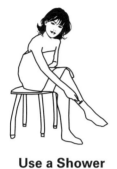

**Use a Shower
Stool**

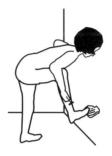

**Use a Raised
Foot Receptacle**

head [454] or on a pole [455] in the corner of your shower. This will eliminate neck strain when using these items.

Ladies, if you shave your legs in the shower, sit on a small shower stool [456] or place your foot on a raised foot receptacle [457] to do so. This eliminates the need to bend your neck and body forward.

Rather than bending over to rinse soap off your legs, let the shower do the rinsing work.

If the width of your shower area is so narrow that the shower curtain often clings to your body, causing you to have to twist to detach it, purchase a curved shower rod [458] that widens your shower area by holding the shower curtain further away.

DRYING YOUR HAIR

Drying your hair has a couple of potential neck hazards. One is that people with long hair often like to wrap their wet hair in a towel on top of their head after washing it. The problem with this is that the weight of the towel and its awkwardness—and your reaction to its awkwardness—can strain your neck.

Another hazard is using a handheld hair dryer to dry your hair. This can strain your neck and shoulder muscles because you have to raise your arms and bend your neck. Instead, if possible, use an electric hair dryer that has a hood

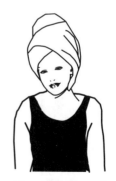

**Head Wrapped
in Heavy Towel
Causes Neck Strain**

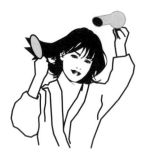
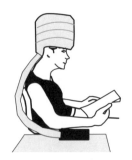
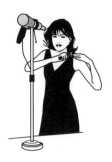

**Incorrect Use of
Handheld Hair Dryer**

**Use a Hair Dryer
with a Hood**

**Use a Hands-Free
Hair Dryer Stand**

to place over your hair or purchase a hands-free hair dryer stand [459] to hold your handheld hair dryer in a position above your head.

And, as another reminder, if you have long hair, do not quickly turn your head to sling your hair back out of your face while drying it. This action may strain the muscles and sprain the joints of your neck.

DRYING YOUR BODY
When drying yourself, avoid using an extra-long absorbent towel. The effort this requires can strain your neck. Instead, use smaller towels.

APPLYING MAKEUP
Ladies, when you apply makeup, sit or stand up straight and use an adjustable mirror [460] that can be pulled close to your face. Or, place a separate mirror [461] (one other than the mirror over your sink) against the wall so you can get close to it without having to bend over the sink. Another

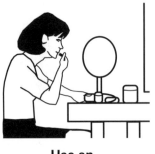
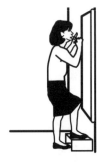

**Use an
Adjustable Mirror**

**Use a
Wall Mirror**

option is to use a magnifying mirror[462] so that you do not have to be so close to it. The point here is to avoid bending your head and neck forward to get close to the mirror, as this will strain your neck and cause your head to misalign forward. As a general rule, always look straight ahead at the mirror and avoid bending or twisting your neck.

And, a quick reminder: If you stand up to apply your makeup, always prop one foot on a small step stool[406] or open a cabinet door and place one foot on the bottom edge of the cabinet. Look straight ahead at the mirror. This posture will maintain the curves of your neck and back and will take the stress off your neck.

TOILET ACTIVITIES
Toilet Paper Holders
Though this may sound a little funny, try not to twist your neck and back to reach for toilet paper, as this movement can hurt your neck. If the placement of your toilet paper holder requires you to twist, take as much toilet paper as you need before you sit down or put the toilet paper roll in your lap. Better yet, use a freestanding toilet paper holder[463] and place it in front of you and to one side.

Flushing a Toilet
Again, do not twist to flush the toilet. Always have your face and toes pointed toward whatever you are about to do. The most neck-friendly way to flush a toilet is to stand up, turn around, place your feet facing the flushing handle, bend down by pushing your buttocks backward and bending your knees, and keep your back and neck straight. Supporting yourself with one hand, reach out with the other and push the handle.

Beauty Salons and Barber Shops

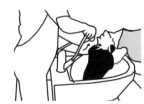

Dangerous Neck Posture When Washing Hair

No doubt you have experienced the neck pain that comes from visiting your hairstylist. Never let your beautician lean your head backward to wash your hair. This practice can lead to more than a painful neck strain—if you bend your neck more than fifteen degrees

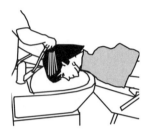

Correct Neck Posture When Washing Hair

backward during shampoos, it can cause a stroke! This is sometimes called "beauty parlor stroke." Instead, keep your neck straight and lean forward into the washing and rinsing bowl.

The neck-aids and neck-appliances described in this chapter can be ordered through your family chiropractor or from the Neck and Back Products store at **www.NeckAndBackProducts.com** or call toll-free **1-800-882-4476.**

7

Child Care Activities That Place a Strain on Your Neck

Being pregnant and caring for small children can offer many neck-straining opportunities. You will need to be especially careful of neck injuries during pregnancy and for the initial six months after delivering a child. The reason is that when you are pregnant, your body produces a hormone called Relaxin that relaxes your ligaments. Your ligaments remain relaxed (stretched) for six months after your child is born, thus making your neck more vulnerable to injury during this time.

After your pregnancy, you may be so busy at times taking care of your child that you do not correct any postural faults that developed when you were pregnant. As your ligaments re-tighten, they solidify any postural problems you have at that time—possibly for the rest of your life. Therefore, pay special attention to your posture after pregnancy so that your ligaments tighten while you are holding yourself in proper spinal alignment.

CARRYING A BABY

Always carry your baby as close to your body as possible, preferably against your shoulder. To illustrate the incorrect way of carrying a baby, pick up a bowling ball and hold it out at arm's length. Then try to hold it there for five minutes. You will not be able to do it. You will strain yourself. Then hold the bowling ball next to your body. This you will

be able to do almost effortlessly without straining yourself. The bowling ball weighs about the
same as a baby, and when you carry it next to
your body it produces less strain.

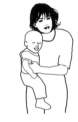

**Carrying a Baby
Incorrectly**

Carrying your child on one hip raises your
hip and forces upward your shoulder on the
side that carries the baby. This causes your
mid and lower back to sag in one direction
with your neck kinking back in the opposite direction, placing a strain on your neck.
If you need to carry a child, either on your
shoulder or on your hip, alternate from one
side to the other so that neither side takes all
of the strain.

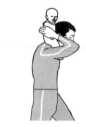

**Avoid Carrying
Baby on Shoulders**

Likewise, carrying a child on your shoulders pushes your neck forward, injuring your
neck. Avoid this!

Feeding a Baby

When breastfeeding or bottle-feeding a baby, instead of rounding your
upper back to reach the baby, bring the baby up to you. If you are breastfeeding, turn the baby so that its stomach is against your stomach.

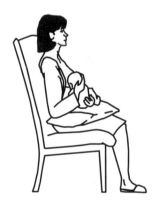

**Correct Nursing Posture
Sitting**

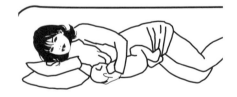

**Correct Nursing Posture
Lying Down**

Burping a Baby

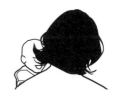

Be careful when holding, rocking, or burping your child over one shoulder. You want to avoid bending your head to the side too far because this position will strain your neck.

**Avoid Neck Strain
When Burping Baby**

Lifting a Baby

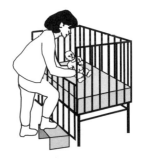

Bending over to lift a child out of a low crib can strain your neck muscles. If possible, and if safe for the baby, raise the crib mattress to waist level to reduce frequently bending your neck forward.

Additionally, lifting your baby out of a crib with your arms stretched out in front of you places a lot of strain on your neck. A more neck-friendly practice would be to place one foot on a step stool [406], put the side of the crib down,

**Taking Baby
Out of Crib**

lean your forearms on the edge of the side of the crib, bring your child as close to your body as you can, and then lift using the strength of your arms and legs.

Many new mothers develop pain in their wrists that many times extend to their thumbs. During the later stage of pregnancy, tendons and joints become lax to give women extra flexibility during birth. Immediately after birth, the tendons and muscles are suddenly required to pick up and

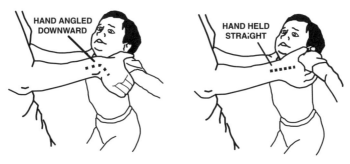

Avoid Wrist Strain

put down a heavy baby many times a day. In doing so, many women let their wrists bend toward the ground with their fingers angled downward, over-stretching the lax tendons over the bones of the wrists. This over-stretching and irritation causes an inflammation of the wrist and thumb tendons, called tendonitis. The answer to this painful problem is to keep your hand in correct alignment with your forearm. This follows the adage "If you don't bend it, it won't hurt."

Bassinets

Raise your child's bassinet to your waist level. You may want to safely secure the bassinet to the top of a chest of drawers or bureau. When you are changing or playing with your baby, place your foot on a step stool [406] to maintain the curves of your back and neck. If you do not have a step stool, remove the bottom drawer of your chest of drawers and place your foot in that space.

The Height of Your Baby-Changing Table

The pad on top of your baby-changing table should be at the height of your waist. If you do not have a waist-high changing table and if it is safe for your baby, raise the baby's crib mattress to waist height, or place your baby on top of a chest of drawers or bureau. You could also place the baby on your bed and kneel on the floor next to him or her to change the diaper.

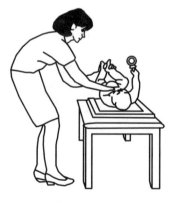

**Incorrect
Baby Changing Height**

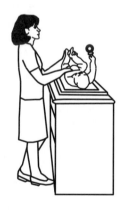

**Correct
Baby Changing Height**

BATHING YOUR BABY

For its first six months, bathe your baby in the kitchen sink or in a portable baby bathing tub that is placed on the kitchen or bathroom counter rather than bending over a tub, straining your neck.

If your kitchen countertop is too low, purchase an over-the-sink shelf[464] and place your child's bathing soap, wash clothes, etc., on this higher level. By raising the height of your baby's bath items, you reduce the amount of forward bending of your neck that will be necessary.

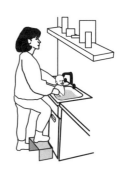

Washing Baby in Sink

Baby Carriers

The best way to carry a newborn who weighs less than ten to fifteen pounds is in a "baby sling"[200] that hangs in front of your body.

The "baby sling" is a versatile and hands-free method of carrying a baby. However, your baby may become uncomfortably hot inside the sling. Therefore, be aware of the temperature outside. While carrying your baby in the sling, always make sure its breathing is unobstructed. Additionally, never run or jog with a baby in a sling or any type of baby carrier—the jarring motion can injure a child's spine or brain.

The best way to carry heavier babies is in a backpack baby carrier[201] where the weight of the baby is more evenly distributed over your back. A front baby carrier[202], a different type of infant carrier, places the baby on the front of your chest, also distributing the weight correctly.

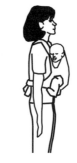

Front Baby Carrier

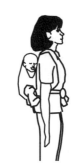

Back Baby Carrier

When you carry a baby in a baby sling or backpack-type carrier, make sure you do not lean your upper body backward or forward to compensate for the extra weight you are carrying; doing so will force you to counterbalance yourself by bending your neck in the opposite direction, straining your neck.

Placing a Small Child into an Automobile

Lifting and twisting to place a child into a child restraint seat can strain your neck. As soon as possible, teach your child to get into the seat him- or herself.

It is best to use a child safety seat that doubles as a baby carrier[203]. These child safety seats are composed of three sections: a baby carrier, a stay-in-the-car base, and a baby stroller. This type of seat eliminates much of the twisting, reaching, and straining that would occur if you were to place a safety seat in the vehicle first and then place your baby in it. If you use a baby carrier that is not made up of three sections and has to constantly be placed in and out of your vehicle, it will be too heavy and awkward and you run the risk of straining your neck each time you place your child into your vehicle or move your child out of the vehicle and into a stroller. Therefore, to reduce the stress to your neck muscles, buy and use a child safety seat that can be separated into a baby carrier, stay-in-the-car base, and stroller.

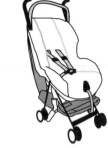

Baby Carrier/Stroller/ Car Seat Combination

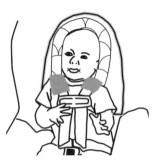

Circular Head Support for Baby

If you transport your child in more than one family vehicle, purchase a child safety seat[203] with a detachable baby carrier and a stroller for each vehicle and leave the base of these seats affixed to your car seats and the stroller section in your vehicles' trunks. Detaching, moving, and reattaching the old-fashioned child safety seats produces more strain on your neck than does placing a child in the seat.

For protecting your child's neck from strain, purchase a circular head and neck support[204] to place beneath your child when he or she is in the baby carrier portion of the child safety seat. This support is a semicircular pillow that is placed around your infant's head to prevent it from flopping to one side.

INFANTS

Always place your infant (weighing up to twenty pounds) in the backseat of your vehicle in a child safety seat that faces backward. Avoid placing your infant in the front seat, because the rapid expansion of an air bag could severely or fatally injure your child. In an emergency, if you must place an infant in the front seat, disconnect the passenger-side air bag and face the child safety seat toward the seatback.

For your infant's neck health, be careful when lifting or lowering your baby into the baby carrier portion of a child safety seat or stroller. Too often parents pull infants up or reposition them by pulling on their arms. This strains the infant's shoulders and neck and allows its head to flop around, possibly misaligning the baby's neck.

Also, always place the child safety seat as far away from the vehicle's doors as possible. Expanding side-door air bags can be fatal if the child safety seat is placed too close to the doors or if the child is allowed to sleep leaning against the door of the vehicle. Adjust the child safety seat so it is firmly attached to the car seatback. Make sure to securely buckle the seat belt and shoulder harness.

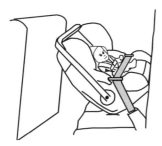

**Correct Position
of Infant in Vehicle**

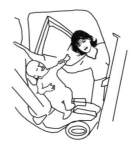

**Don't Lift Child by
Pulling on Arms**

Safety Hints

- The National Highway Safety Administration reports that 85 percent of child seats are installed incorrectly. Correctly installing a child seat can reduce the chance of your child's death in an automobile accident by 75 percent. To make sure that your child safety seat is properly attached, go to a safety seat inspection facility. To locate a facility in your area, call 866-SEAT-CHECK (866-732-8243) or visit *www.seatcheck.org*.

- If you primarily use the backseat of your vehicle to transport children, consider choosing a vehicle without side air bags.

- If you have an automobile with only front seats, consider purchasing one without a front seat passenger–side air bag or with a passenger-side air bag that can be turned off.

CHILDREN WEIGHING TEN TO TWENTY POUNDS

For children weighing ten to twenty pounds, place the child in a rear-facing child safety seat that is placed in the backseat of your vehicle. Make sure the back of the child safety seat does not lean toward the seatback. This position will allow your baby's head to flop forward, injuring its throat and neck. The back of a correctly placed child safety seat should slant toward the dashboard at a forty-five degree angle. First, secure the base of the safety seat, then place your child in the baby carrier, and then sit on the seat next to the child safety seat base and place the baby carrier into the base.

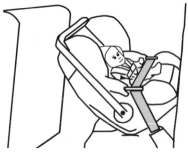 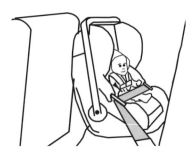

Correct Placement of Child Safety Seat   **Incorrect Placement of Child Safety Seat**

To best protect your neck, follow these steps:

- Hold the baby carrier (with your child in it) against your chest.

- Facing the rear seat of the vehicle, lean into the vehicle while simultaneously placing your foot inside on the rear floor. At this point, most of your body should be inside your vehicle, and you should be squatting slightly without twisting your torso.

- Move your body as far into your vehicle as you can while keeping your head, neck, and back straight.

- Get as close to the child safety seat base as possible.

- Then move the baby carrier an additional foot to place your child into the base of the safety seat.

- The harness straps should be placed at or below shoulder level.

- Be careful when picking up your child when he or she is in a baby carrier; it is easy to forget how heavy a small child is.

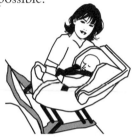

Lifting Child in a Child Safety Seat

CHILDREN WEIGHING TWENTY TO FORTY POUNDS

Once your child is more than a year old, or weighs over twenty pounds, place him in a three-piece child safety seat, previously described, in which the base is securely fastened to your vehicle's backseat. The child safety seat should be placed in a face-forward position and leaning backward at a forty-five-degree angle. Never place a child in a safety seat that sits the child in a straight-up position, as this position can cause the baby to drop its head forward, straining its neck and cutting off its airway. The harness should be placed at or below shoulder level.

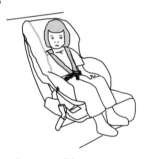

Correct Placement of 40+ lb Child in Vehicle

Purchase a larger child safety seat when your child's head reaches the top of the seat. A child safety seat that is too small can injure your child.

Remember, as soon as possible, teach your child how to get into the seat alone.

CHILDREN WEIGHING MORE THAN FORTY POUNDS

Children over forty pounds usually have outgrown child safety seats. At this stage, place your child face forward in a vehicle safety approved child

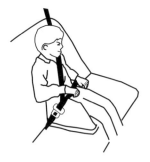

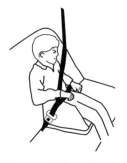

**Incorrect Placement
of Seat Belt**

**Correct Placement
of Seat Belt**

booster seat [205] in the backseat of your vehicle and away from the side doors. Placing a child over forty pounds or from ages four to eight with a height less than four-feet-eight-inches in a child booster seat reduces the child's risk of injury by 50 percent.

Child booster seats vary in appearance, but usually look like the booster chairs that are used in restaurants to elevate a child to table level. The booster seat raises the child to a level where adult seat belts fit properly across his or her shoulders and lap.

The best child booster seat is one that is secured by an adult lap-shoulder seat belt system. If you must use a child booster seat that is only secured by a lap belt, get a booster seat with a plastic shield that fits between the seat belt and the child's abdomen. A lap-belt-only securing system, without the shield, can injure your child's abdominal muscles or internal organs in an automobile accident.

Continue using a child booster seat until your child is big enough to be protected solely by adult seat belts, usually around eight years of age, above forty pounds, or more than fifty-seven inches in height (i.e., when the across-the-shoulder seat belt crosses your child's chest, not his or her neck). If the seat belt crosses your child's neck, severe neck and throat injuries can occur, or even death, if you have an accident.

A SIDE NOTE ABOUT CHILDREN'S NECK HEALTH:
Do Not Have Your Children Work Too Hard ... Too Young

Quite often when children are in their adolescent and teenager years, they experience rapid growth. When we see tall young bodies, we automatically think they are strong, but this is not true. Tall does not equal strong. As a teenager, tall just means the child has had a growth spurt. The muscles of adolescents and teenagers are actually weak because they are still developing. Muscles still in their development stage can be easily strained, and immature ligaments are easily sprained if they are used to lift items that are too heavy.

The spinal bones of adolescents or teenagers are also very weak because they have not had enough time to solidify into a strong bone yet. The spinal vertebrae at this age, instead of being hard like an adult's bone, are as soft as a sponge. Heavy lifting at this age can easily crush these vertebrae, resulting in your child's having a rounded mid back for the remainder of his or her life.

When adolescents and teenagers lift objects that are too heavy, the weight of the object pushes down on their spines and can impede or cut off the blood supply to their vertebrae and discs. Children at this age are continuing to grow taller and can easily outgrow the blood supply to their spine if it is reduced in any way. If this happens, the result is that the vertebrae collapse or crush. And, once a vertebra collapses (crushes), it never recovers.

You have heard the saying, "Hard work never hurt anyone." A doctor would never say those words, because doctors have seen the damaging effects of heavy lifting and hard work done by bodies not yet mature enough to handle it. Let your children do the work of an adult when they become adults. Until then, help them develop strong, straight, normal, healthy spines.

The neck-aids and neck-appliances described in this chapter can be ordered through your family chiropractor or from the Neck and Back Products store at **www.NeckAndBackProducts.com** or call toll-free **1-800-882-4476.**

8

How Cars and Trucks
Hurt Your Neck

Men drive an average of forty-four miles a day, while women drive thirty-four miles a day on average. Most of us drive in vehicles that do not protect us from vibrations and that are deficient in postural design. These deficiencies, along with our posture when driving or riding in a vehicle, produce tension and fatigue in our neck, upper and lower back.

The car or truck you drive has a direct effect on the health of your neck. Repeated jolts, jars, and vibrations of a moving vehicle can sprain your neck just as badly as a fall can sprain your neck. People who spend half their time driving a vehicle are three times more likely to herniate a disc (remember that a disc is a type of ligament, and any injury to it can be called a sprain). The reason: road vibration. Imagine what a series of "hammer blows" could do

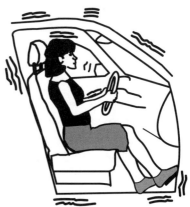

Vibrations of Vehicle

to your neck and you will have an idea of what the vibrations from a car ride can do.

This chapter offers tips for avoiding activities and situations that produce neck strains while you are driving or riding in a vehicle. For a complete discussion of how to "neck-proof" your car or truck, see Chapter 13.

Types of Vehicles

The first step to reducing the strain caused by driving is, if you can, to get a car that fits your body size. You do not want to have to bend your neck into an awkward position when entering, exiting, loading, unloading, or riding in it.

Typically, it is best to drive a large, heavy car or van instead of a mid-size or compact vehicle. Larger vehicles absorb the jolts, jars, and vibrations created when the vehicle is moving and prevent you from being tossed around easily. Smaller, lighter vehicles produce more vibrations and "road jarring" than larger vehicles do.

Low, sporty cars or cars with small doors may force your neck into an awkward, uncomfortable position as you enter or exit them. Each time you are forced to bend or twist your neck getting in or out of a vehicle, a tremendous strain is placed on your neck muscles. This, of course, leads to neck pain.

A four-door automobile is preferable, but a van or Sport Utility Vehicle (SUV) is recommended for those who frequently need to load or unload children or cargo. In fact, vans are more neck- and back-friendly than most other vehicles.

However, there are big differences among the various models of vans and SUVs. Some vans and SUVs are built primarily for commercial use (i.e., hauling cargo, etc.). Others are built with family or passenger usage in mind. These vans and SUVs may look alike, but you will need to test-drive them to notice the difference.

Vans or SUVs built for family or passenger use will vibrate less and have a smoother, less jarring ride. Conversely, the commercial models vibrate more, produce more road jarring, and have a rougher ride. When shopping for a new vehicle, always test-drive as many vans and SUVs as possible to select the one with the least vibrations and the softest, least jarring ride.

Trucks are stiffer, do not absorb impacts as well, and produce more vibration and road jarring than automobiles. In fact, the more you can avoid riding in them, the better off your neck will be!

If you do not frequently have to load or unload children or items into the backseat of your vehicle, a two-door vehicle with big doors is recommended. The larger the doors, the more space you will have in which to maneuver when entering or exiting the vehicle. The greater the space, the easier it will be to maintain good posture and keep your neck safe.

If possible, drive only vehicles that have an automatic transmission and power steering. These features will minimize the stretching, twisting, and pulling that your neck will be subjected to while you drive.

If getting in and out of your vehicle or driving causes you neck pain, your neck needs a different type of vehicle!

Lastly, the most neck-friendly automobile is the Volvo. Its Whiplash Protection System (WHIPS) has been proven to reduce head and neck injuries by 49 percent. Volvo is the "neck-safest" automobile in the world.

Vehicle Seats

Sports cars often have seats so low that they force your legs straight out in front of you. This causes your lower back to bend backward and your neck to bend forward, straining it. Vehicles with low seats are also more difficult to get in and out of, creating additional strain to your neck muscles.

Conversely, a vehicle seat can also be too high. Some trucks and vans have seats too high to allow a comfortable entrance or exit. However, your seat should be high enough to keep your knees elevated at least one inch above your hip joints.

PROPER SEAT POSITION

If your seat is too far back, you will have to bend your neck forward and round your shoulders in order to drive, thus straining your neck and upper back muscles. Position your seat so that the front of your body is approximately twelve inches from the steering wheel.

You want to sit close to the foot pedals and adjust the vehicle's seat so you can maintain your

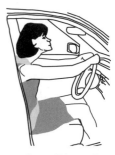

**Seat Placed
Too Far Back**

upright posture while placing your feet on the floor. Make sure your heels are on the floor and your toes are within easy reach of the foot pedals. Doing so will help you avoid stretching to use the pedals. You should be able to work your pedals with just your feet, not your legs, hips, or back.

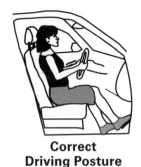

**Correct
Driving Posture**

THE BOTTOM OF THE SEAT

The bottom part of your vehicle's seat should be medium firm. If your seat is too soft, your body will slump, which, as you know, will force your neck to bend excessively forward, straining your neck muscles.

If the bottom of your seat is too deep from front to back, it will force your lower back into a backward curve, which will force your neck to bend forward, straining both structures. If the front edge of your seat rubs the back of your knees, your seat is too deep from front to back. There should be a four-inch space between the front edge of your car seat and the back of your knees. If the front edge of the seat places pressure on the back of your lower thigh, the back of the car seat is too low. You should be able to easily slip two fingers between the back of your lower thigh and the front edge of your car seat.

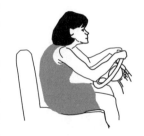

**Too-Deep Car Seat
Causes Poor Posture**

THE SEATBACK

If your car seat does not allow your neck muscles to relax, neck strain will be the result. The back of your car seat should be firm, have a good lumbar (lower back) support, and be angled fifteen degrees backward. A fifteen-degree angle and a lumbar support help maintain your spinal curves, allowing your back and neck muscles to relax.

There should be a space at the bottom of the seatback that allows your buttocks to protrude slightly beneath it or into the seatback. If your seatback does not have this feature, the back of your buttocks will be pushed forward by the seat, forcing your lower back into a slumped, rounded position and your neck into an opposite bending position, straining it.

If your seatback does not have a good built-in lumbar support, add one to your seat to support the contours of your body. A lumbar support for automobiles [100] should be adjustable to your body size and shape and should have straps or a cover made of non-slip material to help it stay in place on the seat. Make sure your lumbar support pushes the small of your back slightly forward.

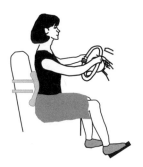

Adjustable Lumbar Support for Automobiles

When sitting in your vehicle, push your buttocks all the way to the back of the seat and tighten the seat belt to keep your hips from sliding forward.

SPORTS CAR SEATS

If you drive a true sports car, the safety of your neck was probably not your highest priority in choosing your vehicle. Nevertheless, we chiropractors must advise: "Avoid sitting in a car with bucket seats, or racing seats." These seats are too hard and usually do not provide adequate lower back support. If you must sit in a vehicle equipped with these seats, place a feather pillow (not foam-rubber) on the seat bottom. This extra cushion helps absorb some of the bouncing and jarring of the moving vehicle and thus helps to protect your

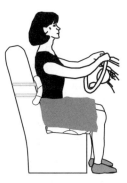

Add Pillow to Car Seat

neck. Also, place a lumbar support for automobiles [100], mentioned previously, on the back to support the curve of your lower back because when your lower back curve is maintained in the proper position, the curve of your neck will also be correctly positioned.

If your vehicle has improper seat bottoms or backs, see Chapter 13 to learn how to modify the seats to properly support your body.

Getting in and out of a Vehicle

The simple steps of opening a vehicle's door or getting in or out of a vehicle can cause neck strain. The following instructions will teach you how to get in and out of a vehicle with little or no strain to your neck.

There are two ways to enter a vehicle: backward or forward.

The following instructions are for getting into a vehicle from the driver's side. When you enter a vehicle from the passenger's side, follow the same instructions but use your opposite hand and ignore the steering wheel instructions.

GETTING INTO A STANDARD-SIZE AUTOMOBILE OR TRUCK

Open the driver's door all the way. Make sure it is completely open and not going to swing shut on you while you are getting into the vehicle. Push the seat of your vehicle all the way back. If you have a tilting steering wheel, tilt it all the way up and out of the way. If your vehicle has a telescoping steering wheel, push it all the way in to make additional room for your entry.

Stand with your back to the door opening, facing away from the vehicle. Back up until you feel the back of your legs against the vehicle. Your feet should be approximately twelve inches apart with one foot slightly ahead of the other. Place your left hand on the metal post that is between the front and back window on the left side of your vehicle or on the top of your vehicle's seat. Place your right hand on the steering wheel, on the roof of your vehicle, on the post in front of your vehicle's door, or on any other structure that will safely support your weight.

While holding on to these support structures, bend your knees and gently back into your vehicle, leading with your buttocks while lowering your upper back and neck forward. Then, lower your buttocks down onto the seat of your vehicle.

Once your buttocks are on the seat, reposition your right hand to the right side of your vehicle's seat or armrest, and reposition your left hand

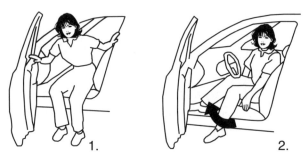

Getting into Standard-Size Vehicle

onto the left side of your seat. Then, keeping your legs together, bend your knees further, lift your feet off the ground, and rotate your body and both legs into your vehicle (like spinning a log on its end). Continue rotating your body and legs into your vehicle until you are in a forward-facing position, with both legs in your vehicle. Then, extend your feet to the pedals.

At this point, slide your buttocks to the back of your seat. Readjust your vehicle's seat so that your lower back is supported against the lumbar support that is built into the back of the seat or against a lumbar support you have added to your vehicle. Your knees should be slightly bent and slightly higher than your hip joints. Then, readjust your steering wheel and fasten your seat belt. Now, you are ready to drive. Perform this maneuver without twisting your neck or body.

GETTING INTO A LOW AUTOMOBILE OR TRUCK

Many automobiles, especially sports cars, are built stylishly close to the ground. These low vehicles are rarely designed for tall individuals. When a vehicle's ceiling is too low for someone tall, the person will be forced to crunch down in the seat and place his or her head in a harmful head-forward posture. This posture produces neck and upper back pain. And, since these cars are so difficult to get in and out of, it is best to avoid them altogether. However, in case you want to keep your sports car, here are some instructions that will help to protect your neck in low cars and trucks.

In order to get into the driver's seat of a low vehicle, open the driver's door all the way and make sure it will not swing shut on you while you are getting in. Then, reposition the steering wheel as previously described. Next, face the open door, place your left hand on the left side of

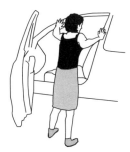

**Getting into
Low Vehicle**

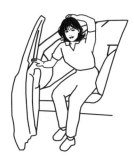

**Protect Head When Entering
and Exiting Vehicle**

the doorframe and place your right hand on the upper right-hand portion of the post between the front and back seat or top of the car seat for support. Then squat to seat height and lean your upper body forward, reposition your left support hand onto the steering wheel and your right hand onto the car seat. At this point, bend forward more, keeping your neck straight, and slide your head, neck, and body into the vehicle, moving forward toward your rearview mirror. Once in the vehicle, keeping your neck straight, slide your hips onto the seat and your feet under the steering wheel. Then sit up straight, bringing your head, neck, and body to their normal positions.

If your vehicle is not too low, and you do not have to crawl into it as described, put one of your hands on top of your head to prevent hitting it on the doorframe. A sudden hitting of your head can misalign neck vertebrae.

GETTING INTO A TALL AUTOMOBILE OR TRUCK

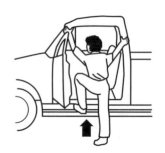

Open the driver's door all the way and make sure it will not swing shut on you while you are getting in. Then, reposition the steering wheel as previously described. Facing the open door, grab the inside of the doorframe of the driver's door with your left hand and the steel post behind the driver's window with your right hand. Pull yourself upward

Getting into Tall Vehicle

with your hands while you climb into the automobile or onto the steps of the truck. Then crawl into the vehicle in the same manner as you would to get into a sports car with low seats.

GETTING OUT OF A STANDARD-SIZE AUTOMOBILE

To get out of the car, first move the front seat of your automobile as far back as it will go. If you have a telescoping steering wheel, push it all the way in. If you have a tilting steering wheel, push it up and out of the way. Then open the door all the way, making sure the door is not going to swing back and hit you when you are getting out of the vehicle.

Place your right hand on the steering wheel and your left hand on the outside top of your car seat or on the post between the front and back windows—or if your automobile has a handle between the front and back windows, grab this handle with your left hand. Lift both legs off the floor-boards. Then, keeping your head, neck, and body straight, and again using the strength of your arms, spin your entire body and legs, as a unit, on your buttocks (like spinning a log on its end) until you are facing the open door. Swing your feet and legs outside the car door at the same time.

Still using the strength of your arms, slide your buttocks to the outside edge of your car seat. Then, place your feet on the ground twelve inches apart, one foot slightly in front of the other, and secure a good footing on the ground.

At this point, reposition your right hand on the doorframe of your car door and your left hand on the post between your front and back window for better support. Keeping your back straight and your head facing forward, lean your body slightly forward from your hips and pull your feet backward toward the vehicle in order to establish better balance. Using the strength of your arms, pull yourself into the standing position, while simultaneously pushing upward with your thigh and calf muscles and reaching for the sky with the top of your head. Your back and neck muscles should not be used at all during this maneuver.

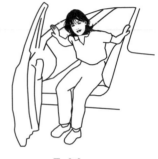

**Exiting a
Standard-Size Vehicle**

If the roof of your vehicle is too low, once you have your feet firmly on the ground and have repositioned your right hand on the doorframe and your left hand on the post between your front and back door, you will have to lean slightly backward, keeping your

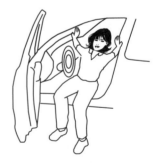

**Forty-Five-Degree Angle
Exiting Technique**

head facing forward and your back straight. Then using your arm muscles, slowly pull your body through the door opening, buttocks first. Once your head has cleared the top of the door frame, use the strength of your arms to pull yourself into a standing position, while simultaneously push-ing upward with your thigh and calf muscles and reaching for the sky with the top of your head. There is no completely neck-friendly way to exit a car with a too low roof, but by using this maneuver you will greatly decrease the risk of injury to your neck or back.

GETTING OUT OF A LOW AUTOMOBILE

Again, begin to get out of the car by first opening the door and pushing the seat all the way back. If you have a telescoping steering column, push it all the way in. If you have a tilting steering wheel, tilt it up and out of the way. Placing your left hand on the steering wheel and your right hand on the car seat, turn your body to the right (left shoulder toward the steering wheel). At the same time, lean your upper body into your automobile

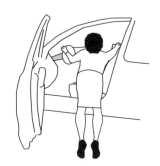

Exiting a Low Vehicle

toward the rearview mirror. When your body is leaning approximately forty-five degrees, slide your legs and buttocks out of the car until both feet are on the ground. At the same time, walk your body out of your automobile with your hands and push your body outward. When your head gets outside, reposition your hands onto the doorframes on either side of the door, stand up, keeping your neck and back straight.

GETTING OUT OF A LARGE (TALL) AUTOMOBILE OR TRUCK

Use the "exiting backward technique" when getting out of a tall vehicle where you have to step down to reach the ground.

Slide your seat all the way back. Adjust your steering wheel so that it is out of the way. Then, placing your left hand on the steering wheel and your right hand on the seat, turn your body to the right (left shoulder toward the steering wheel). At the same time, push your upper body into the vehicle toward the rearview mirror. When your

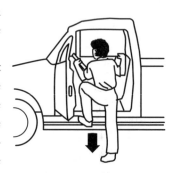

Exiting a Tall Vehicle

body is leaning into your vehicle, slide your legs and buttocks out of the vehicle. Place one foot on the step of the vehicle. Your next step is either onto a lower step or onto the ground. Keep both hands on their supports until your feet are secure on the ground. Then, walk your way out of your vehicle with your hands.

If you have a very tall vehicle, you will need to change the supports for your hands while exiting. Grab the vehicle doorframe in front of the driver's door with your left hand and the post behind the front window with your right hand. It is very important to maintain a three-point contact throughout your descent—two hands on a support and one foot firmly on a step or on the ground.

Correct Driving Posture

Whenever you drive a vehicle, pay attention to your sitting posture. Sit up straight and relax, always maintaining the natural curve of your neck. Poor driving posture, including slouching, will strain your neck muscles and sprain your ligaments.

Instructions for sitting correctly in a vehicle are:

- Sit up straight, or lean slightly backward without bending your neck. Do not lean to either side.

- Face straight forward with your eyes straight ahead.

- Position the top of the headrest at the same height as the top of your head.

- Make sure your head is no farther than two inches from your headrest.

- Rest your shoulders comfortably on top of your rib cage. Do not lean them forward or backward.

- Keep the front of your body approximately twelve inches from the steering wheel.

- Bend your arms at the elbows with your hands at the nine o'clock–three o'clock position on the steering wheel.

- Rest your elbows on the armrests.

- Sit all the way back in the seat with your buttocks fitting under the seatback.

- Make sure your lower back is slightly arched forward and is supported by the lumbar support of the seatback.

- Your knees should be slightly higher than your hip joints.

- Make sure the back of your lower thighs are 1 to 1½ inches above the front edge of your car seat.

- Make sure the backs of your knees are four inches in front of your vehicle's seat.

- Place the heel of your right foot comfortably on the floor of the vehicle with the ball of your right foot on the foot pedals.

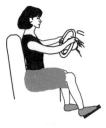

**Correct
Driving Posture**

The Steering Wheel

DISTANCE FROM THE STEERING WHEEL

When you drive, your arms should be slightly bent. A straight-arm posture will strain your neck muscles.

If your seat is too far back, you will have to stretch forward to grasp the steering wheel, which will force you to bend your neck forward in order to drive. This posture will strain your neck. Make sure your body is pushed against the seatback to prevent you from slouching. Also, if your seat is too close to the steering wheel, an expanding air bag could injure you.

Again, the general rule of thumb is that, to maintain good posture, your body should be approximately twelve inches from the steering wheel.

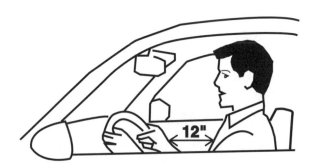

Chest Twelve Inches from Steering Wheel

GRASPING THE STEERING WHEEL

Holding the wheel at the ten o'clock–two o'clock position will cause you to round your shoulders and crane your neck forward, producing a strain of your shoulder and neck muscles. Instead, as noted, grab the steering wheel at the nine o'clock–three o'clock position. This allows your arms and shoulders to rest on your rib cage and allows your neck muscles to relax.

Be sure not to grip the wheel too tightly, as this will tire your neck, shoulder, and arm muscles.

Headrests, Armrests, and Seat Belts

HEADRESTS

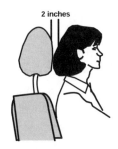

2 inches

Always keep your car's headrests in the up position. This is a real safety issue. It is actually safer to have no headrests than headrests in the down position because a headrest in a down position can act like a fulcrum, producing a more severe injury in an accident.

Set the top of your headrest as high as the top of your head and within two inches of your head. This will reduce your chances of a whiplash if you have a rear-end collision.

Head Two Inches from Headrest

Add-on headrests [101] are available for people who are too tall to be protected by standard headrests, and to close the gap between the head and headrest for people who have a stooped posture or a head-forward posture that results in their head being held more than two inches forward of the headrest.

ARMRESTS

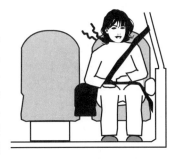

Using an armrest while driving will reduce fatigue of your neck and shoulder muscles. Without an armrest, or by using an armrest that is too low, the weight of your arms will pull down on your neck, straining your neck muscles. The armrest should be tall enough to support your elbows and forearms without your having to lean side-

Too-Low Armrest Causes Neck Pain

ways. Leaning sideways to use an armrest will increase the stress on your neck, straining it.

SEAT BELTS

When first sitting in a vehicle, place your buttocks firmly against the back of the seat, and then tightly fasten your three-point seat belt. This will keep your hips from sliding forward. A three-point seat belt is the combination of an across-the-lap seat belt and an across-the-shoulder seat belt, and is by far the safest type. Relying solely on a lap belt will not prevent your head and chest from hitting the steering wheel if you are involved in a front-end accident.

Do not place your across-the-shoulder seat belt across your neck or under your arm. A seat belt placed across your neck can kill you in an accident and a seat belt placed under your arm can wring your spine in an accident, severely injuring it.

CAUTION: Do not assume that because your vehicle has air bags you do not need to use a seat belt. You do! In fact, air bags create another need

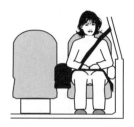

**Correct
Armrest Height**

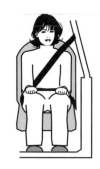

**Correct
Placement
of Seat Belts**

for seat belts. If you have an accident and are not wearing a seat belt, the air bags—which expand at 230 mph—may project you over the seat and out the back window.

The use of seatbelts has reduced serious injuries by 75 percent. For your safety, please always wear a seat belt when driving.

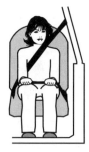

**Incorrect Placement of
Seat Belt - Across Neck**

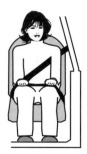

**Incorrect Placement of
Seat Belt - Under Arms**

Do Not Sit on an Object

Never sit on your wallet or any other object because it will push one of your hips upward, which will force your lower spine to one side. Your upper spine and neck will then be forced to lean in the opposite direction. This awkward posture will strain your back and neck.

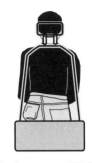

Sitting on a Wallet

Do Not Lean on the Window Frame

Leaning on the window frame while seated in a vehicle forces your lower back to sag in one direction while your upper back and neck sag in the opposite direction, straining your back and neck muscles.

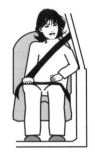

Leaning on Window Frame Causes Harmful Posture

Turning Your Neck While Driving

Avoid rotating your neck to look over your shoulder when backing up a vehicle or checking for traffic. This posture wrings your neck. Instead, when it is safe to do so, use your rearview and side-view mirrors to accomplish this task.

If you must turn to see behind you, use your whole spine. You have joints all the way down your spine—use them all. First, turn your lower back, then mid back, and lastly your neck. This way, your neck only has to turn one-third as far and you will be able to look right out the back of your vehicle without hurting yourself.

If you have difficulty backing up your vehicle because your neck is stiff, purchase an easy-to-attach, inexpensive radar-like device [102] that would audibly warn you of people or

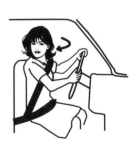

Avoid Excessive Rotation of Neck

items that are behind your vehicle. By using this type of device, you may not have to turn your neck as far when backing up your vehicle.

Also, do not quickly twist your neck to make lane changes, or stretch and twist your neck while driving. These activities can strain your neck.

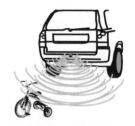

Radar Device That Alerts You to Objects Behind Your Vehicle

Using a Cell Phone While Driving

Though extremely popular, talking on a cell phone while driving is a serious hazard for several reasons. First, bending your head and neck to the side to hold the phone next to your ear will place your neck under significant stress. Worse yet, each year 1.5 million crashes and 570,000 injuries result from people using cell phones while driving. To keep your neck (and the rest of you) safe from injury, only use a cell phone when you are not driving a vehicle.

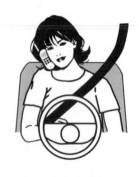

Use of Cell Phone Causes Neck Strain

Red Lights

Avoid getting too close to a red light. If you are too close, you will have to bend your head and neck forward and then raise your chin up to see the light, straining your neck.

Accelerating and Braking

Accelerating or braking too quickly will push and pull on your neck, producing

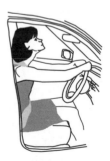

Getting Too Close to a Red Light Causes Neck Strain

a neck problem—and possibly whiplashing your neck.

Also, sudden acceleration from high-powered engines will sprain the necks of unsuspecting passengers. Be conscious of the health of your passengers and avoid being a passenger with anyone who drives like a "jack rabbit" (i.e., with fast starts and stops).

Rough Roads

**Avoid Fast
"Starts" and "Stops"**

The micro-trauma (shocks, bumps, etc.) caused by riding on rough roads can injure your neck. Therefore, avoid driving on rough roads whenever possible.

Driving Long Distances

Vehicle vibrations are a primary cause of ruptured discs. To avoid creating disc problems, try not to drive or ride in a vehicle for more than two hours per day.

If you must drive long distances, stop every hour and walk around for five to ten minutes and do gentle range-of-motion neck exercises (described in Chapter 16).

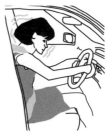

Sleeping in a Vehicle

Never sleep sitting up in a vehicle without a proper travel pillow [420]. The bobbing and flopping of your head to the side will strain your neck.

**Sleeping in Vehicle
Causes Neck Strain**

Loading Items into an Automobile

When you load packages into your car, reduce the weight of your packages into many smaller, lighter loads, if possible. Heavy loads pull on your neck; light loads do not.

If you drive a two-door automobile, put your packages on the front seat or in the trunk. Do not put anything in the backseat because it is too difficult to get anything in and out without straining your neck. If you have a four-door automobile, there is no problem placing packages and other items in the backseat. When loading items onto a car seat, place them close to the door for easy lifting.

If you drive a station wagon, van, or SUV, place your packages close to the rear door for easy access in and out.

If you need to carry items in the trunk of your car, place the objects in the trunk as close to the back bumper as possible. This will reduce your need to bend forward.

Neck-friendly ways of placing children into automobiles are discussed in Chapter 7.

Lifting Objects out of Your Vehicle

An important guideline for reducing neck strain no matter what you are doing is: Do not be lazy! Take the extra steps necessary to keep your neck pain free. This applies to lifting objects out of your vehicle. Do not attempt to unload packages that are in the passenger seat of your car while you are sitting in the driver's seat. Get out, walk around to the other side, and then unload the car safely. Otherwise, you will twist your neck. Likewise, do not try to lift packages that are in the backseat of your vehicle when you are sitting in the front seat. Get out, open the back door, and then lift.

Avoid overstretching when attempting to grab an object that is placed too far away from you. The overstretching can strain your neck. If a package is not within close reach, get into your vehicle and pull or push the item toward the edge of the seat, then lift.

If you have packages in the backseat of a two-door automobile, get out of your vehicle, slide your front seat up, then—keeping your head, neck, and body straight—enter the vehicle and kneel on the backseat to grab the object. Then, slide the object to you, hold it close to your body, and then lift it.

LIFTING LIGHT ITEMS OUT OF A VEHICLE'S TRUNK

When picking up small or light objects off the floor of the trunk, place the hand that you are not going to use to grip the item on your car fender or on the edge of your trunk to support yourself. Then, keeping your head

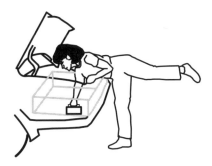

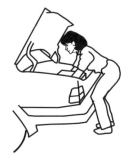

Correct Light Lifting Technique   **Correct Heavy Lifting Technique**

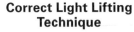

up and your neck and spine in a straight line, bend straight over from your hip while keeping the leg on the side of your gripping hand slightly bent. Simultaneously, let the leg and foot on the side of your support hand come off the ground, keeping the leg aligned with your upper body. Grasp the item you intend to lift using the hand on the side of your standing leg, and bring the item close to your body. Then, lift the item by dropping your leg on the side of your support hand while simultaneously raising your body—keeping your head, neck, body, and leg in a straight line.

The counterbalancing of your body with your leg will allow you to come back up straight without using the muscles of your neck or back.

LIFTING HEAVIER ITEMS OUT OF A VEHICLE'S TRUNK

To safely lift heavy items from the trunk, follow these instructions. Open the trunk, stand as close to the rear bumper as you can, place your feet under the bumper, bend your knees slightly, and push them against the rear bumper. Then, keeping your neck and back straight, bend forward by pushing backward with your buttocks and then leaning forward. Grab the object that is to be lifted and bring it as close to the edge of the trunk as possible. Lift the item and place it on the ledge of the trunk as an intermediate step. Then, slide the object onto your thighs, pull it toward your chest, and lift.

Preparing for a Collision

If you have been warned of an impending collision (e.g., you hear people yelling, the screeching of tires, etc.) and you have time to prepare yourself for the impact, do the following:

Look straight ahead—not at the passengers in your vehicle. Do not turn your head because an impact can wring your neck. Straighten your arms and grip the steering wheel with both hands, hard. **CAUTION:** Never place your hands over the air bag module cover. The expanding air bag can break your arms. Push yourself all the way back in your seat and place your head firmly against the headrest. Brace one foot on the floor and, with the other foot, put total pressure on the brake pedal. Make your body stiff and tense and brace yourself for the impact.

The neck-aids and neck-appliances described in this chapter can be ordered through your family chiropractor or from the Neck and Back Products store at **www.NeckAndBackProducts.com** or call toll-free **1-800-882-4476.**

9

Recreational Activities
That Can Injure Your Neck

Many recreational activities require you to bend and twist your neck and thus strain your neck muscles and sprain your ligaments. It may seem like the list of harmful activities is long—it is. But even if you still choose to participate in these activities, it benefits you to know the problems they cause so that you can more consciously protect your neck when doing them.

Going to the Movies

Sitting in the front rows of a movie theater will force you to raise your head upward sharply to view the screen, forcing your head into the head-forward posture and straining your neck muscles. Always sit farther back; after all, you cannot see the whole screen from that close anyway! Always sit in the middle section of a movie theater because sitting in the side sections will force your neck into a twisted position for a long period of time.

Sports

Be careful when doing any sports activities or aerobic exercises that may strain your neck. Whenever a sports activity pulls excessively on your neck, stretching or ripping of the muscles can occur. Sports and other recreational activities that frequently pull on your neck muscles include riding on roller coasters, rowing or using rowing machines, gymnastics, javelin throwing, wrestling, bumper cars, weight lifting, weight training, and aerobics.

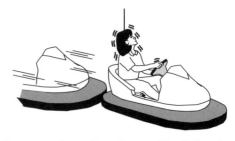

Bumper Cars Can Cause Neck Strain

IMPACT SPORTS

Impact sports can strain your neck muscles and sprain the joints of your neck. The impacts or falling that occurs in basketball, football, lacrosse, hockey, boxing, pole-vaulting, trampoline, rodeo riding, martial arts, rugby, bumper cars, water skiing, snow ski-ing, ice skating, soccer, and diving can injure your neck.

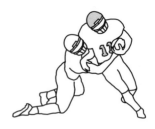

One particularly dangerous maneuver in soccer is "heading" the ball. This is when the ball has been kicked in the air and a player hits the ball with his or her head to help advance the ball. This provides a significant impact on the head and bones of the neck.

Avoid Impact Sports

SPORTS THAT CAUSE MICRO-TRAUMA

As you know, micro-trauma, or many little jolts, to your neck can cause a neck injury. If you have a straightened or reversed spinal curve in your neck, the discs will be more easily damaged by micro-trauma. Sports that produce micro-trauma include race-walking, running, jogging, ballet, aerobic dancing, break dancing, tap dancing, rope skipping, horseback riding, trail-bike riding, bicycle racing, snow skiing, water skiing, snow-mobiling, and tobogganing.

There is a difference in the amount of micro-trauma produced by walk-ing, race-walking, jogging, and running. Walking, which allows your head to stay balanced on top of your spine, produces almost no micro-trauma because your knees and ankles prevent most of the micro-trauma from reaching your spine. Race-walking and jogging produce the most micro-

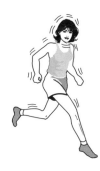

Running Causes Micro-Trauma

trauma because your heels hit the ground, causing jars to the spine. In running, your toes and the balls of your feet hit the ground, not your heels. Most of the jarring micro-trauma is therefore absorbed by your feet, ankles, and knees—with little force hitting your spine.

Even so, run only on smooth, familiar surfaces, cinder tracks, grass, or soft ground, rather than on asphalt or cement. The softer the running surface, the less likely any micro-trauma will affect your neck. And, if you wear bifocals or trifocals, where it is necessary to tilt your head to see the ground ahead, consider using single-vision glasses instead.

BOATING

The repeated jolts, jars, and vibrations of a boat ride can do more damage to the discs of your neck than will a car ride. Imagine what the repeated vibrations of a jackhammer would do to your neck, and you will have an idea of what a boat ride can do. To protect your neck, only ride in a boat if the water is smooth. Rough waters will repeatedly jolt, jar, pull, and vibrate your neck, possibly causing injury.

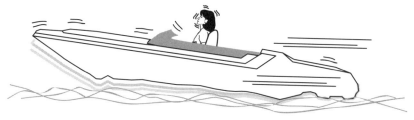

Boating Causes Micro-Trauma

TWISTING SPORTS AND EXERCISES

Sports and exercises that involve twisting have a tendency to strain your neck muscles and misalign your spinal vertebrae. This type of sport and exercise includes baseball, tennis, basketball, soccer, football, bowling, racquetball, hockey, lacrosse, handball, squash, figure skating, golf, gymnastics, high-impact aerobics, and volleyball.

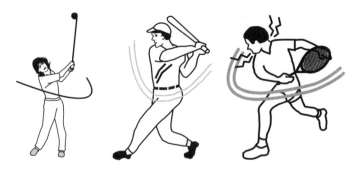

Avoid Twisting Sports

The twisting effects of golf can be minimized by not turning your neck to the side while it is bent forward (in the backswing) and shortening your backswing. Also, reduce the time you let your head hang forward; instead, step back slightly to address the ball while keeping your neck in a more neutral position.

SPORTS AND EXERCISES THAT PLACE YOUR NECK IN AWKWARD POSITIONS

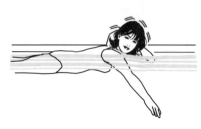

**Rotation Strain
Caused by Swimming**

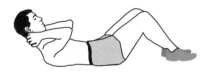

**Improper Sit-Ups
Cause Neck Strain**

As you know, awkward body positions can strain your neck muscles, misalign your spinal vertebrae, and jam the facets in your neck. Sports and exercises that place your neck in an awkward position include cycling, sit-ups, figure skating, wrestling, backpacking, certain yoga positions, and certain swimming strokes (e.g., the butterfly, breaststroke, and crawl). All of these activities can place stress on your neck.

When performing sit-ups, do not use your hands to support, pull on, or place counter-pressure on your head and neck. Instead, cross your arms over your chest.

SPORTS THAT CAUSE EXCESSIVE BACKWARD BENDING OF YOUR NECK

Backward bending of your neck jams the facets at the back of your neck, pinches nerves, and stretches your neck muscles. Sports that produce this

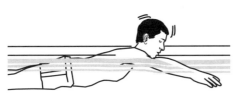

type of backward bending include gymnastics, tennis (e.g., when serving), javelin throwing, shot-putting, pole-vaulting, weight lifting, breaststroke or the butterfly stroke when swimming, and wrestling.

Avoid Backward Bending of Neck

SPORTS THAT WORK ONE SIDE OF YOUR BODY

One-sided sports pull on and over-build the muscles on one side of your neck, straining your neck muscles and possibly misaligning your spinal vertebrae. Examples of one-sided sports are fencing, bowling, racquetball, golf, javelin throwing, baseball, softball, tennis, handball, squash, table tennis, and badminton.

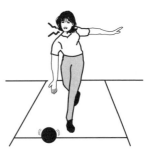

**Bowling Can Cause
Neck Strain**

GOOD SPORTS

Yes, there are sports that do not injure your neck! Gentle sports such as most swimming strokes, bike riding, hiking, and walking are the least likely to cause neck problems.

Yoga and Pilates are excellent exercises to loosen tight muscles and increase your range-of-motion. However, avoid any position that over-bends your neck forward (e.g., shoulder stands) or backward (e.g., back-bends and headstands) as these positions can strain your muscles and put pressure on the discs of your neck.

The best exercise is swimming, with the exception of the particular strokes mentioned already—those that require you to arch your neck backward or over-rotate your head to the side, then straight, then

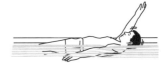

Good Swimming Posture

to the side again. This repetitive motion can strain your neck. The most neck-friendly type of swimming is the backstroke, which allows you to relax your neck while letting the water support the weight of your head.

Diving is another story altogether. Hitting the water with your head can sprain your neck. See the earlier description about impact sports.

While bike riding is an excellent exercise that does not strain your neck, you must ride the correct kind of bicycle. If you use a stationary bicycle,

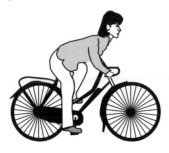

**Low Handlebars
Cause Neck Strain**

make sure the seat and handlebars are at the proper height for your body. You should be sitting in an upright position, not bending over to reach the handlebars. The same applies to a regular bicycle. Avoid bicycles with curled-down handlebars that force you into a forward-leaning posture. This bent-forward posture of your head and neck and rounded shoulders produce a strain to your neck muscles. Use handlebars that allow you to sit up straight. Put a mirror on your helmet or bicycle so you can see behind you without having to twist your neck. It is also wise to ride a bicycle that has wide tires rather than standard-size tires. Wide tires produce less vibration and thus reduce the micro-trauma to your neck. Riding on smooth terrain also reduces micro-trauma.

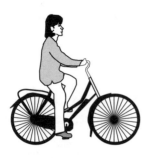

**Correct Posture
While Bicycling**

Other sports that are not injurious to your neck are fishing, scuba diving, and ballroom dancing.

10

Long-Distance Travel Activities That Can Strain Your Neck

If you have traveled much at all, you know that leaving the comforts of your home and familiar surroundings can be physically taxing. Carrying luggage, getting in and out of planes, trains, and automobiles, and sleeping in a bed other than your own can cause stress and strain on your neck. This chapter covers some basic ways to reduce neck strain when you travel.

Your Luggage

PACKING

Avoid twisting, stooping, or over-reaching when packing or unpacking luggage. To avoid unnecessary bending, it is a good idea to place your luggage on a table, bureau, or bed when packing.

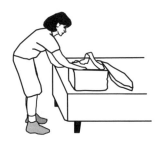

Place Suitcase on Bed

TYPES OF LUGGAGE

As we all know, packed luggage can get very heavy and be difficult to carry. If possible, buy lightweight luggage with wheels for ease in moving and carrying. Larger wheels are good because they prevent your luggage from

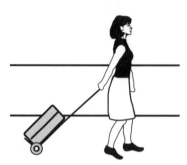

Portable Luggage Carrier

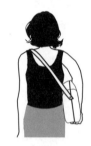

**Correct Placement
of Shoulder Strap**

twisting sideways when you are pulling it. If your luggage is difficult to pull, you will more likely strain your neck and shoulder muscles trying to do so. Collapsible luggage carriers with wheels [800] make getting luggage from one place to another easy. If your luggage does not have wheels, rent a rolling cart at the airport or get someone else, such as a porter, to carry your luggage for you.

When possible, avoid taking carry-on luggage, especially carry-on luggage that has a shoulder strap. If you must take carry-on luggage, only use the type that rolls on wheels. If you use a bag with a shoulder strap, you will have to elevate your shoulder on one side (lowering the opposite shoulder as a result) to prevent the strap from slipping off and sliding down your arm. This posture pulls on your neck and shoulder muscles, straining them, and can misalign your neck vertebrae.

If you wish to use a shoulder strap for security purposes, place the strap over your head and across your body, and place the luggage under one arm to help carry it. The point is to not have to carry the entire weight with only one side of your body. To further relieve your neck and shoulder muscles, alternate the carry-on bag from one side to the other.

AMOUNT OF LUGGAGE

When traveling, consider taking two smaller suitcases instead of one large, heavy one. This way you can distribute the weight between both arms. If you only pack one heavy suitcase, one side of your body ends up carrying the entire load, straining your upper back and neck muscles.

Do your best to keep the number of your luggage pieces to a minimum to avoid excessive lifting. If you travel on business, send your documents

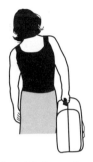

**Avoid Carrying
Heavy Suitcases**

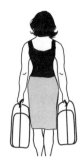

**Carry
Two Smaller Suitcases**

and books ahead via fax, email, or commercial carrier. By easing your load in this way, you avoid the strain the weight of these items can have on your neck.

Storage Bins

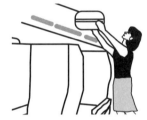

The effort required to place your luggage in the overhead compartments of buses, planes, and trains strains your neck, upper back, shoulder, and arm muscles. If you must take carry-on luggage, store it under your seat. If your carry-on is a garment bag, hang it in the closet.

**Avoid Lifting Luggage
Above Shoulder Level**

Airplane and Bus Seats

Airplane and bus seats usually push your head and neck into a bent-forward position. They also cause your lower back to bend backward, straining your neck and lower back. To counter the strain on your lower back and neck, place a small airline-type pillow at your lower back and a travel pillow [420] around your neck to correct your posture.

TRAVEL PILLOWS

Because airplane and bus seats provide poor neck support, they allow your head to flop from side to side or nod forward. When traveling by plane or bus, always bring a travel pillow [420] with you. These pillows are usually made of foam rubber and covered in fabric. They are also ideal for high–backed chairs and settees that do not give ad–equate neck support. **CAUTION:** If your travel pil–low is too large behind your neck, it will force your head forward, placing a strain on your neck muscles.

INFLATABLE TRAVEL PILLOWS[801]
These pillows support your neck when you are at–tempting to sleep while traveling. They fit neatly into your pocket or purse when deflated and can be in–flated easily when needed.

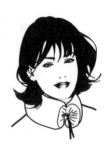

Travel Pillow

Hotel Rooms or Strange Surroundings

Always bring your air pillow [417] with you when you are going to sleep in strange surroundings. Substandard pillows will strain your neck and ruin your sleep.

If you forget your air pillow, place your travel pillow behind your neck when you sleep.

The neck-aids and neck-appliances described in this chapter can be ordered through your family chiropractor or from the Neck and Back Products store at **www.NeckAndBackProducts.com** or call toll-free **1-800-882-4476.**

11

Strenuous Activities
That Can Strain Your Neck

M any of the strenuous activities discussed in this chapter are mentioned to various degrees throughout this book. Lifting, carrying, pushing, and pulling all strain the body and have great potential to damage your neck when done improperly. In this chapter, we will look at each of these activities and discuss the most neck-friendly ways of doing them.

Lifting

The heavier an object is, the more dangerous it is to lift. Lifting pulls on your neck muscles, straining them. Lifting something heavy strains them more severely. Be careful, and always think before you act! Your chances of injury increase dramatically with every pound you lift.

When you have to lift an object, your nose and your toes should face the object. Keep your head up to maintain your normal cervical curve. Do not bend your head forward or let it hang forward when lifting because you will add extra strain to your neck. Proper lifting technique is obtained by placing your feet at least twelve inches apart, bending downward by pushing your buttocks backward and bending your knees, not your back. Never lift anything with your back rounded, by bending from the waist, or with your legs straight, because you will strain your back and neck muscles. Always maintain the curves in your spine when lifting, especially the inward curve of your lower back. When your lower back curve is inward, the curve in your neck will be too. Keeping your back, head, and neck in proper alignment while lifting means there will be less stress to your neck.

Once your posture is in correct alignment, then make sure you have a good grip on the object you are going to lift. If it slips, you will jerk to grab it—and that is when you will hurt your neck.

Always bring the weight to be lifted as close to your body as possible. A ten-pound weight held at arm's length will feel like you are holding seventy to one hundred pounds. If the weight is held close to your body, ten pounds will only feel like ten pounds. Lifting objects at arm's length strains your neck and upper back muscles. And, whenever you lift an object away from your body, it increases the stress on your lower back. As you know, anything that is stressful to your lower back is automatically stressful to your neck. Lift the object with your head and neck in their normal position, using your legs and arms to lift it. Your leg and arm muscles are the strongest muscles in your body and can lift better than your back can.

GUIDELINES FOR LIFTING

- Divide large, heavy loads into multiple small loads.

- Think before you act! Check out the object to be lifted. For example, loose materials in a box can shift and throw you off balance, straining your neck.

- Always face the object to be lifted. Never twist your body while lifting. Always keep your "nose between your toes"—with both your nose and your toes facing the object to be lifted. This posture stops your body from twisting or leaning as you lift. If you find that your nose is no longer between your toes as you lift, this means your body has rotated or is leaning to the side. If so, stop your lift and repeat it the correct way.

- Always bring the object you are lifting close to your body.

- Do not jerk the load when you are lifting; jerking can hurt your neck muscles.

- Avoid lifting objects above shoulder level. Lifting heavy objects above this point can cause neck strains, sprains, and disc problems.

- When you lift an object from waist height, such as when moving it from one desk to another, make sure your legs, shoulders, hips, and back all turn as a unit, with your feet moving first.

- Use lifting aids whenever possible. If you have to lift something heavy, use a mechanical device (e.g., an electric garage door opener), rather than lifting it by hand, or get someone to help you lift it.

LIFTING TECHNIQUES

The heavier the object, the greater the strain it puts on your neck when lifted improperly. However, even the lightest objects can easily injure your neck when proper lifting techniques are not followed. When you have to lift an object, regardless of how much or how little it weighs, put the least amount of strain on your neck by using one of the following lifting techniques.

Side Lift

This technique is used for lifting heavy objects with one hand, such as a toolbox.

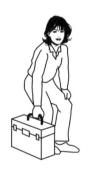

Position your body so that the side from which you will be lifting is as close as possible to the object. Bend your knees, keep your neck and back straight, squat down to get a good grip on the object, for support put your non-lifting hand on the thigh opposite the item to be lifted, then smoothly straighten your legs while pushing upward with your support hand. If you simply grab the object to be lifted and then forcefully lift it, you will strain your neck and shoulder muscles.

Side-Lifting Technique

Golfer's Lift

This technique is used for lifting small items off of the floor or out of the trunk of a car without expending too much energy or straining your back.

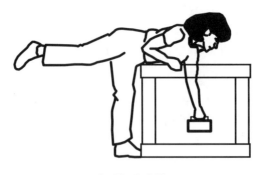

Golfer's Lift

Place your support hand on a fixed object for support, then place all of your weight on the leg opposite your support hand while keeping your neck and back straight. Bend forward from your hips, keeping your head and spine in a straight line, and extend backward the leg on the side of your supporting hand to counterbalance your weight. With your free hand, grab the object to be lifted and pull it up while simultaneously lowering your leg.

Olympic Lift

This technique is used for lifting heavy objects off of the floor using both hands.

Straddle the item to be lifted. **NOTE:** If the item is too big to be straddled, then it is too big for one person to safely lift. Your feet should be apart, about the width of your hips, with one foot slightly forward of the other. Try to keep the object to be lifted between your legs. Bend

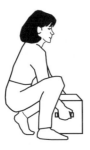

**Straddle Items
to Be Lifted**

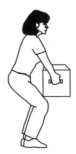

Olympic Lift

down by pushing backward with your buttocks and bending your knees. Do not bend from the waist. Keep your head up, shoulders back, and spine straight or with your lower back slightly arched.

Securely grip the object to be lifted to avoid any slipping. If the object slips, you will jerk to grab it, and that is when you will hurt yourself. Tuck your elbows and arms in and pull the object as close to the middle part of your body as possible (the farther away the object is from your body, the more stress you will place on your back and neck).

Lean back to balance yourself. Lift the object using the strength of your legs in as smooth a motion as possible. Straighten your knees to come to a standing position.

If the object is very heavy, prop it on your thighs as an intermediate step, then lift to your chest, and then the rest of the way up.

Straight Back Lifts

This technique is used for lifting something over a barrier, such as getting groceries or heavy trash bags out of the trunk of a car, a baby out of a crib, and so on. It is the least preferable of all types of lifts because it places the most stress on your neck and back.

First, get close to the object. Press your (slightly bent) knees against the barrier for support. Keep your back and neck straight. Bend downward by pushing your hips backward. Do not arch your back because you will arch your neck at the same time, straining it. Get a good grip on the item to be lifted. Check out the object to be lifted—loose items can shift while being lifted, throw you off balance, and strain your neck. Next, pull the

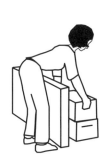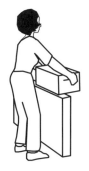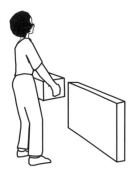

Straight Back Lift

item as close to you as possible. Place the item on the barrier to reposition it for carrying, and again bring the item close to you. Then stand up by pushing up with your leg, hip, and back muscles. Reverse this procedure when you need to put an object down over a barrier.

Below Shoulder-Height Lift

This lifting technique is used when placing an object on a surface that is between waist height and shoulder height.

Face the object to be lifted. Place your feet twelve inches apart, with one foot slightly behind the other. Keeping your head up and maintaining your neck and back curves, bend your knees to reach the object you want to lift. Check out the object to be lifted—loose items can shift while being lifted, throw you off balance, and strain your neck. Bring the item to be lifted close to your body while also keeping your elbows close to your body. Then, use your arm and leg muscles to lift and push the item upward onto the surface.

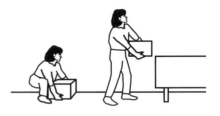

Below Shoulder Lift

Above Shoulder-Height Lift

This lifting technique is used when it is necessary to place an object on a surface above your shoulder height. In general, try to avoid lifting objects above shoulder level since this can easily cause neck and back problems.

Face the object to be lifted. Place your feet twelve inches apart, with one foot slightly in front of the other. Keeping your head up and main-

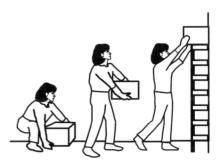

Above Shoulder Lift

taining your neck and back curves, bend your knees to reach the object you want to lift. Then, grab the opposite corners of the box/container/object to be lifted. Test the weight for unevenness or loose contents and find the center of gravity of your load. Any sudden repositioning of the object's weight can strain your neck. Lift the object to between waist and chest height. Keeping your back leg bent, put the bottom edge of a free corner of the object against the top edge of the surface you want to place it on. Shift your hands underneath the box, keeping your elbows in. Then, push the item onto the surface using your leg and arm muscles while simultaneously shifting your weight forward as you lift and shove the object onto the surface.

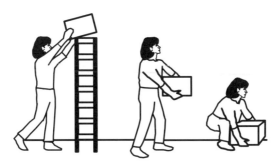

Retrieving Objects Above Shoulder Height

Retrieving Objects from Above Shoulder Height

When retrieving an object from a surface that is above your shoulders, keep your back leg bent to absorb the weight. If possible, test the weight of the object. Slide the object to the edge of the surface. Then, keeping the object against the edge of the surface, slowly slide the load down to your mid body. Then, shift your weight backward as you pull the item off of the surface. Avoid arching your back because that will also arch your neck, straining it.

Women's Lifting

In addition to the lifting guidelines as given in this chapter, women are advised not to wear tight skirts or high-heeled shoes while lifting, as these make it impossible to balance and position yourself correctly and safely.

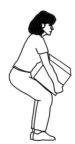

Putting Objects Down

If you are carrying a heavy weight at waist level or above, put it down by sliding it down your leg.

Slide Heavy Objects Down Leg

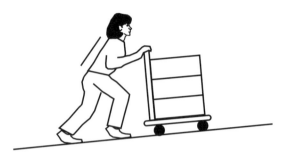

Push Heavy Objects

Pushing

Pushing an object is easier and safer than pulling it. You can also push twice as much weight as you can pull; therefore, make it a habit to push instead of pull.

When pushing an object, keep your knees bent, your back straight, your head up, and your arms close to your sides. Your feet should be placed twelve inches apart with one foot slightly in front of the other. Lean into the object, and then push off with your back leg. Push with your legs and arms and take short steps.

Pulling

Try to avoid pulling anything. And certainly never jerk while pulling something. The natural tendency will be to stand flat-footed and to yank, relying solely on your upper back and neck muscles; for example, as when attempting to pull open a window that is stuck. This action pulls on your neck muscles, straining them.

Proper Pulling Technique

If you must pull on something, follow these guidelines. Keep your back straight. Place your feet twelve inches apart and one foot slightly in front of the other for balance. Keep your elbows close to your sides and maintain your spinal curves. Shift your weight backward when pulling. This posture is similar to a water skiing posture. Get your balance. When you lean back, push forward with your front foot. If you notice your back beginning to round or your shirt tightening, you are pulling incorrectly.

When pulling a cart toward you, make sure you keep your feet clear of the cart's wheels.

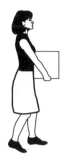 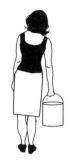 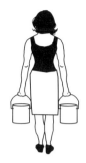

**Carry Heavy Objects
at Waist Level**

**Don't Carry
Heavy Objects
in One Hand**

**Carry Two
Small Loads**

Carrying

Ideally, all loads to be carried should be at waist level and close to your body. Carrying items in this manner produces very little stress to your arms, neck, and back.

The farther away from your body you carry an object, the more pressure you put on your discs, and the more strain you will place on your neck and back muscles. For every pound that is held one foot in front of you, fifteen pounds of pressure occurs in the discs and muscles of your spine. Thus, if you hold a twenty-pound object one foot in front of you, it will transmit a 300-pound load to the spine's discs and muscles. Also, the closer an object is held to the body, the more evenly its weight is distributed over the spine, pelvis, and legs.

Avoid carrying anything in one hand or under one arm. If you are carrying a bag, toolbox, etc., shift it from one hand to the other.

Do not carry "lazy man" loads. Carrying too much at one time will strain your neck and back muscles.

Better yet, if you have to carry a heavy object, ask for help. If help is not available, do not carry the item in one load; separate it into smaller loads in order to reduce the weight of each load and, if necessary, make several trips. This will reduce the straining of your neck, shoulder, and arm muscles. It is wisest to have two small loads of equal weight, one in each hand, to distribute the weight evenly to both sides of your body. This weight balancing will help you avoid straining your muscles.

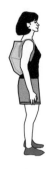

**Carry Objects
in Backpack**

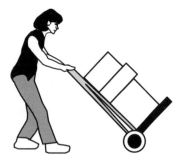

**Transporting Heavy
Objects on a Dolly**

CARRYING AIDS

Instead of carrying a heavy object in your hands, place the object in an ergonomically correct backpack [449] that distributes the weight over both your shoulders and upper back.

When carrying heavy items for a distance, use a carrying aid with wheels (e.g., a cart, dolly, wagon, wheelbarrow, etc.). Any heavy item should be transported on wheels, even if you are moving it only a few feet.

A Caution about Backpacks for Children

There is a new and alarming trend occurring: Young children are suffering from more neck and back pain than ever before. Studies have shown that 74 percent of children who use a backpack develop back pain—the cause being backpacks that are too heavy or that are carried improperly (i.e., carried over one shoulder). When a backpack is too heavy, or when the weight is not distributed correctly, muscle fatigue and strain result, which can lead to headaches, neck pain, back pain, poor posture, a head-forward misalignment of the skull, and a worsening of pre-existing spinal problems such as scoliosis.

Unfortunately, children are carrying backpacks that are so heavy that the children look like vertical turtles with shells on their backs. Besides the back and neck strains and the head-forward misalignment and worsening posture, there are long-term effects that may not show up for twenty years after the child quits wearing a backpack. Spinal misalignments, dysfunctional areas of the spine, restricted movement of the spine, headaches, osteoarthritis, and disc degeneration may also occur. Remember

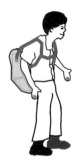

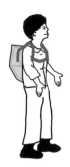

**Incorrect Placement
of Backpack**

**Correct Placement
of Backpack**

the proverb "As the twig is bent, so grows the tree." This also applies to the use of backpacks. Recent research in France has revealed that the longer a child wears a heavy backpack, the longer it will take to correct a deformity of their spine.

Here is how to solve the backpack problem:

- Only let your child carry an ergonomically correct backpack [449].

- Make sure your child's backpack weighs no more than 5 to 10 percent of his or her body weight. **CAUTION:** Adding extra books, electronic devices, and water bottles to a backpack can easily add ten to fifteen pounds.

- Always place the heaviest items in the backpack first.

- Never let your child's backpack hang lower than his or her waist. A backpack that hangs too low will force the child to lean forward while walking, straining his or her neck and back and causing the child's head to misalign forward. If a backpack forces your child to lean forward, it weighs too much.

- A backpack with individualized compartments helps distribute and stabilize the weight better.

- Instruct your child not to carry a backpack on one shoulder. Lugging a backpack around by one strap will force the child to lean to one side, with his or her head and neck leaning to the opposite side, straining the neck and back. Urge your child to wear both shoulder straps.

- Wide, padded straps are better than narrow ones because narrow straps cut into the shoulders, straining the child's neck and shoulder muscles.

- Let your child use only a backpack that is equipped with a hip strap, in order to pull the load tight against the child's body.

- Tighten the shoulder straps to your child's body. If the backpack does not have adjustable shoulder straps, throw it away and purchase an ergonomically correct backpack [449]. Straps that are too loose cause the backpack to be carried too low, or awkwardly, leading to spinal misalignment and pain.

- Consider a backpack on wheels, called a Rolling Backpack [465]. These are much more neck-friendly. The Rolling Backpack is very similar to the wheeled carry-on luggage used on airlines. Some schools require a doctor's note before they will allow a student to use this type of backpack. Call your chiropractor and request a written recommendation for your child.

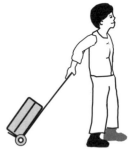

Rolling Backpack

PUTTING ON THE BACKPACK

Finally, instruct your child in the neck-friendliest way to put on a backpack, as follows. Face the backpack, bend at the knees, and use both hands to grasp the backpack. Lift the backpack by using the strength of the legs. Put on one shoulder strap, and then the other.

The neck-aids and neck-appliances described in this chapter can be ordered through your family chiropractor or from the Neck and Back Products store at **www.NeckAndBackProducts.com** or call toll-free **1-800-882-4476.**

Section Three:

Neck-Proofing Your World

12

Neck-Proofing Your Home

Most people's homes are filled with one-size-fits-all furniture and surface areas. Rarely do people buy their furniture or plan the rooms in their home based on what is best for their posture. This is of course understandable. The problem, though, is that when surfaces and furniture do not "fit" the individual's body, the person's body ends up twisting and bending to fit the furniture or surface, usually becoming strained in the process.

People, of course, come in all sorts of shapes and sizes. Children range from one foot tall and upward. Adults range anywhere from three feet tall to seven and a half feet tall. Taller people need higher furniture and work and play surfaces in order to maintain a healthy posture throughout the day. Likewise, shorter people need lower surfaces and smaller furniture that fits them and helps maintain their posture. Children need child-size furniture.

In order to prevent straining and pain in your body—especially your neck—your furniture, kitchen and bathroom surfaces, and all of the tools and appliances in your house need to be adjusted so that when you use them you are maintaining correct sitting and standing postures.

I call this adjusting of surfaces and furniture to keep your neck in its normal relaxed position "neck-proofing." Making your home "neck-friendly" is a simple process that produces instant rewards.

Neck-Proofing Your Family Entryway

Most families enter their homes through the garage or back door. Therefore, place a clothes and hat rack [(466)] at this entrance. The top of this device should be at eye level, with a second clothes or hat rack placed at a lower level for your children. Never stuff clothes or hats into a closet. The pulling, pushing, and straining to find and remove clothes can hurt your neck muscles. Umbrellas should be placed near the exit door in plain view in an umbrella stand or round canister.

Neck-Proofing Your Kitchen

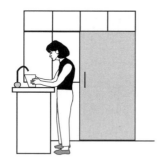

**Correct
"Body to Countertop"
Relationship**

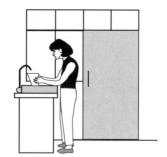

**Add Chopping Block
to Raise Work Surface**

KITCHEN COUNTERTOPS

The proper height for kitchen countertops is at your waist level. If your kitchen countertops are lower than your waist, raise them, if possible. If you cannot raise your countertops, raise your work surfaces instead. You can do so by placing a large, thick chopping block and an over-the-sink shelf [(464)] on your kitchen counter. Do your food preparation on top of the chopping block and place all items such as dishwashing detergent and kitchen tools on the higher level of the over-the-sink shelf. When these items are at the proper height for your body, you will not have to bend your neck to prepare food or retrieve items.

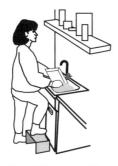

**Use High-Arching
Faucet**

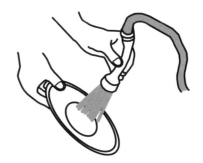

**Use Retractable
Spray Hose**

KITCHEN FAUCETS

Replace your kitchen faucets with a high-arching faucet. Wrestling a heavy pot under a low faucet places an awkward strain on your neck and shoulder muscles. An elevated faucet facilitates your clean-up activities. A retractable spray hose also reduces these strains.

DOORKNOBS AND WATER FAUCET HANDLES

Replace your round doorknobs and water faucet handles with lever handles. Attempting to turn tight, round doorknobs and water faucet handles can strain your neck, shoulder, and arm muscles. Lever-type doorknobs and water faucet handles are much easier to use, and they reduce strain.

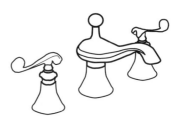

Lever Faucet Handles

KITCHEN UTENSILS THAT STRAIN YOUR NECK

Carpal tunnel syndrome (CTS) is a painful condition of the wrist and hand that primarily affects women. And because the kitchen is primarily a woman's domain, special modifications to kitchen utensils are advised. The typical kitchen knife requires you to bend your wrist forty-five

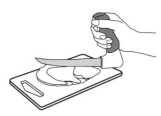

Ergonomic Knife

degrees in order to grasp it. This position of the wrist stretches and inflames the nerves, tendons, and blood vessels that course through a tight tunnel that passes through the wrist (carpal bones). When this occurs, you will strain the contents of your carpal tunnel. Hand and arm pain is the result. Special ergonomic knives[467] and forks will help relieve, prevent, or reduce the discomfort caused by CTS.

KNIFE STORAGE

Storing knives in a kitchen drawer necessitates bending, twisting, and reaching to find the right knife. It also places you in danger of cutting yourself. Instead, hang your knives on a wall-mounted magnetic strip. This method of in-plain-sight knife storage will eliminate all your bending and twisting motions. And, once you wash your knives you can eliminate the drain basket by hanging them up on the magnetic strip to dry.

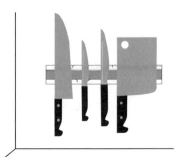

**Wall-Mounted
Magnetic Strip for Knives**

MOST FREQUENTLY USED FOOD PREPARATION UTENSILS

Hang your most frequently used food preparation utensils (e.g., spatulas, whisks, ladles, etc.) from a horizontal rack[468] hung on a wall or from the ceiling directly over your food preparation area. These utensil racks eliminate a significant amount of reaching, bending, and straining.

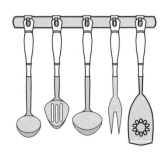

Hanging Utensil Rack

Special, ergonomically designed pots and pans[469] are available. These are more comfortable to use and put less stress on your arms and hands. By minimizing the stress on your arms and hands, you also reduce the stress on your neck muscles.

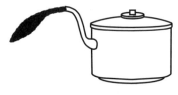

Ergonomic Cooking Pot

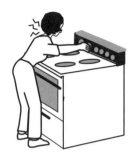

**Overreaching for
Stovetop Controls**

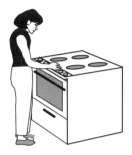

**Stovetop Controls
at Front of Oven**

THE STOVETOP

When it comes time to replace your stovetop, purchase a new one with controls along the front lip or on the side. Stoves with burner controls placed behind the stovetop are ergonomically incorrect, forcing you to reach and strain excessively when turning the stove on and off. Rear-mounted controls are also dangerous. As a side note, whenever you have a stove with burner controls in front or along the side of the stovetop, make sure the controls are the child-proof kind to better protect your family (i.e., the controls are the kind that must be pushed in before they can be rotated).

THE OVEN

The traditional oven is a combination stovetop with an oven at knee level. Ergonomically, this is a back- and neck-straining nightmare. It forces you to bend downward excessively in order to place and retrieve hot, heavy pots and roasting pans.

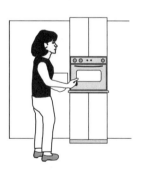

The ideal height of an oven is between waist and shoulder level. This makes lifting objects in and out easy and prevents the arching of your neck backward when placing items in an upper oven.

**Correct
"Body to Oven"
Relationship**

An oven that is too high will force you to strain your neck, especially when you lift items that are heavy. Unless you are building a house, it is likely that your oven is already located too high and cannot be lowered. In

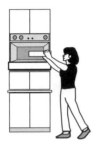

**Oven Placement
Too High**

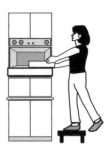

**Use Step Stool to Place
Food in High Oven**

this case, to avoid looking upward, use a stepladder or step stool [406] when placing items in or retrieving items from the oven.

An oven that is too low will force you to bend your upper back and neck too far forward, straining your neck. In this case, squat down with your neck and back straight when moving items in or out of the oven.

Your oven should have a large safety glass and lights that brightly light the interior so that you can check on food without pulling the heavy items out of the oven to view them.

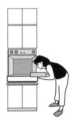

**Oven Placement
Too Low**

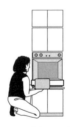

**Squat to Place Food
in Low Oven**

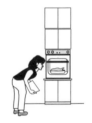

**Oven with Large
Viewing Window**

THE MICROWAVE

To reduce the number of times you have to reach, if you primarily use a microwave to defrost or heat up items, place your microwave atop your kitchen counter next to your refrigerator. If you primarily use a microwave for cooking, place it near your stovetop. Built-in microwaves should be placed between eye and mid chest level.

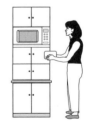

**Correct Height for
Built-In Microwave**

THE REFRIGERATOR

Place your most commonly used food items between eye and waist level with the heavier, bulkier items at waist height. The lighter items should be placed on the higher shelves and the least used items on the lower shelves. This will minimize the awkward bending of your neck and straining when reaching for food items.

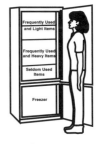

Correct Placement of Items in Refrigerator

The most neck-friendly refrigerator has "French doors"—double upper doors—with the freezer in a separate compartment below. This type of refrigerator allows you to place more of your most commonly used items between eye and waist level. This eliminates most bending over to access frequently used foods.

If a double-door refrigerator/freezer is not practical for you, consider one with a single upper door for the refrigerator section and a single bottom door or drawer for a freezer, as illustrated.

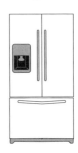

Slide-out shelves, transparent fruit and vegetable drawers are also "neck-friendly" refrigerator features.

Neck-Friendly Refrigerator

THE FREEZER

The most ergonomically correct freezer is a vertical model with many shelves. A horizontal, bin-type freezer requires extensive bending, reaching, and pulling to retrieve items. Each of these activities can strain your neck. The placement of items in the vertical freezer should follow the previously described ergonomic guidelines of food placement in a refrigerator. And the placement of food in a horizontal bin-type freezer or in the freezer section of a refrigerator that has the freezer on the bottom should follow these guidelines. Rarely used food should be placed on the bottom of the freezer and the most commonly used food on top.

THE DISHWASHER

The next time you consider remodeling your kitchen, change the placement of your dishwasher. As you know, dishwashers are usually placed below counter height next to the sink plumbing to facilitate a contractor's or plumber's work. However, no one considered the needs of the person using the dishwasher. A dishwasher should be placed at counter height for ease of loading and unloading. Placing a dishwasher below counter height forces you to excessively bend, reach, and hang the weight of your head and neck forward. All of these actions place a strain on your neck and shoulder muscles.

ERGONOMIC KITCHEN GARBAGE PAILS

For sanitary measures, and to ease bending and straining, use an ergonomic garbage pail [470] that has a foot lever to open the lid and uses gravity to close it. These garbage pails also have handles that make it easy to empty, carry, and clean.

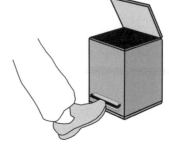

Ergonomically Correct Garbage Pail

KITCHEN PANTRY, DRAWERS, AND STORAGE CABINETS

Using logic in the placement of kitchen items will greatly affect the number of times you have to reach, bend, and stoop to retrieve them. A slight modification of your storage systems will significantly reduce the chances of straining your neck. Most refrigerators and freezers have doors that are designed to open in either direction. If you have to reach around a freezer/refrigerator door to place food items on a kitchen counter,

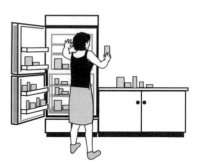

Correct Opening Direction of Refrigerator Door

simply change the direction the door opens to eliminate this awkward movement. The kitchen counter on which you place items taken out of your refrigerator or freezer should be on the side opposite the door hinge. Pull-out cabinet trays, multiple-height Lazy Susans, and theater shelves placed in cabinets will also greatly reduce your reaching and stretching.

To reduce the number of times you must reach for your most frequently used items, such as coffee, sugar, salt, mugs, cereal bowls, and silverware, store them within easy reach of your food preparation counter. Keep your pots and pans near your stove and your knives and dishes near the dishwasher. To reduce reaching, place frequently used items within twenty inches of where you most often need to use them.

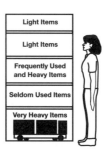

Correct Placement of Items in Storage Cabinet

Store frequently used or heavy items, such as pots and pans, between waist and shoulder height to minimize the need to bend your neck or to reach overhead. The heaviest items should be stored at waist level. By placing heavy items at waist or counter level, you will reduce the straining of your neck when lifting. If you have to store very heavy objects in lower cabinets, store them on a dolly or a cart with wheels so that you can pull them out easily, without straining your neck.

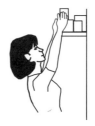

Avoid Reaching Above Shoulder Level

Store light and rarely used items on the highest shelves. When placing items on higher shelves, avoid pushing the items all the way back. Keep them positioned toward the front for ease in grasping them.

Avoid non-transparent storage containers. The prying open of container after container when looking for an item places an unnecessary strain on your neck and shoulder muscles. Transparent storage containers reduce the search for items and the strain of opening multiple containers. A storage area or closet with open shelves and transparent storage containers is ergonomically ideal.

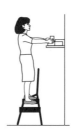

Use Step ladder to Place or Retrieve Items from High Shelves

As a general rule, avoid reaching upward to grasp items on upper shelves. Looking or reaching up places a strain on your neck

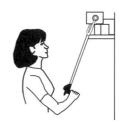

Use of "Reaching Stick"

muscles. Instead, always use a step stool [406], stepladder, or reaching stick [407] to reach higher items.

KITCHEN APPLIANCES

Most kitchen appliances (e.g., coffee makers, knife sharpeners, etc.) are stored under kitchen counters, in cabinets and pantries. Using them requires a lot of walking, reaching, lifting, and pulling. A simple solution to "the appliance mess" is to place them on your kitchen counters beneath your cabinets in appliance garages. At the back of these appliance garages, place electric power strips to plug your appliances into. Whenever you want to use an appliance, open the appliance garage door, pull the appliance out, use it, return it to the appliance garage when you are through, and close the door. Less fuss and strain is the result.

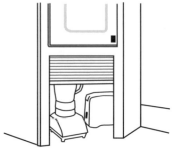

Appliance Garage

PADDED KITCHEN MATS

Small, padded rubber mats are advised for each work area. Most kitchen floors are hard—very hard—such as tile, linoleum, and so on. Prolonged standing on hard surfaces produces foot and leg pain. To relieve this pain, you have to constantly move your legs and body, which also adds strain to your neck muscles.

KITCHEN LIGHTING

Every kitchen should have two types of lighting—ambient and task. Ambient lighting provides general lighting to illuminate a room. Task lighting illuminates specific job areas. Set up your task lights over each specific work area. This lighting is best accomplished by ceiling track lights. Task lights are usually brighter; therefore, add dimmers if these lights are positioned over an eating area. To facilitate finding items, add bright ambient interior lighting to your kitchen pantry and cabinets.

KITCHEN GLARE

White or light-colored kitchen counters and cabinets usually produce glare. Kitchen windows facing south or west produce more glare, especially when the light is reflected off of light-colored counters and cabinets. The more glare produced in your kitchen, the more you must bend over to view whatever you are preparing, thus the more you will strain your neck. To reduce kitchen glare, choose cabinets and counters that are darker and place glare-reducing film on your kitchen windows.

Neck-Proofing Your Family Room and Living Room

FURNITURE ARRANGEMENT

The typical living room or family room has the chairs and sofas arranged "theater-like," in a row facing the television set. While this is ergonomically correct for watching TV, it plays havoc on your neck when you are trying to have a conversation with guests or family members. Can you imagine turning your neck ninety degrees for an hour-long conversation? Neck strain is the inevitable result. The "L" shaped sofa also produces the "wringed-neck" phenomenon. The solution is to set up oval or horseshoe conversation areas in your living room and family room and to use chairs that can swivel for watching TV.

SITTING ON CHAIRS AND SOFAS

Very few chairs and sofas are designed with the support of your neck in mind. They may feel comfortable yet force you to sit improperly, eventually straining and hurting your neck. Sitting, more than all other body positions, places the most stress upon the neck. Therefore, if you want your neck to be pain free, you need to always pay attention to how you are sitting.

One of the reasons sitting is especially offensive to the neck is that most chairs and sofas force you to slouch. Slouching causes your head and neck to bend forward and your shoulders to round. In this position, none of the four curves of the spine can be maintained and, sooner or later, your muscles will become stretched and fatigued—and pain will be the final result. The good news is that any pain produced by slouching will begin to decrease as your sitting posture improves.

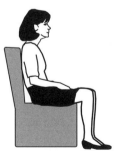

Avoid Slouching

Let us take a look at how you can sit with correct posture to prevent the kind of pain we are discussing. You know your sitting posture is correct when:

- You are sitting up straight, or leaning slightly backward.

- Your head is directly over your shoulders.

- The length of your back is against the chair.

- Your buttocks are as far back in the chair as they can go, slightly beneath the chair back. Once you place your lower back in its proper position, your shoulders, neck, and head will follow, helping to restore the forward curve of your neck.

Correct Sitting Posture

- Your arms are resting on the armrests.

- Both feet are flat on the floor.

- The backs of your lower thighs are one to one and a half inches above the front edge of the seat.

- Your thighs are supported by the seat of your chair.

- Your knees are slightly higher than your hip joints.

FINDING THE CHAIR OR SOFA THAT IS RIGHT FOR YOU

Your personal chair is one of the most important pieces of furniture in your house. It should give your spine enough support for you to relax, watch television, and read for hours. An ideal chair does not force your spine to conform to it, but supports your spine as you adjust or change sitting positions.

Because there is no single chair or sofa that fits all of us perfectly, use the following guidelines to help you find a chair or sofa that is ideal for your body. The first key is to be persistent and not settle for what does not work. Try as many chairs and sofas as necessary before buying the one that fits your body the best. This persistence will pay off big when you consider how much time over the years you will be sitting in that chair or sofa.

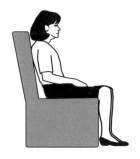 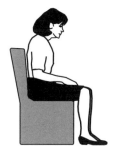

**Oversized Furniture
Causes Slouching**

**Undersized Furniture
Causes Bent-Forward Posture**

FURNITURE SIZE

The size of your furniture is an important part of maintaining a pain-free neck. Although some people love them, oversized chairs or sofas will not give you the lower back support you need and will force you to slouch, automatically causing your neck to bend too far forward, straining it. As mentioned before, this is a leading cause of neck problems. Likewise, a chair or sofa that is too small for you will force you to bend forward, also placing a constant strain on your neck and back.

The more you sit improperly, the more your neck will suffer and progressively worsen. Therefore, only sit in chairs and sofas that fit your body and support your neck and back.

THE CHAIR OR SOFA SEAT

Your chair or sofa seat should be medium-firm and should not sag in the middle. Though popular, soft, overstuffed chairs and sofas are some of the worst culprits for causing slouching and, thus, neck strain. Some chairs or sofas are so soft that the simple act of getting into or out of them will place a strain on your neck, shoulders, and back. As a general rule, if your body indents your favorite chair or sofa more than one inch, the furniture is too soft and will injure your back and neck. To make the seat cushion more firm, you can place a special support board [471] underneath it.

Oversized chairs or sofas often have a seat that is too deep from front to back. The front-to-back depth of the seat is very important when you are trying to prevent neck pain. When you place your buttocks firmly against the back of the chair or sofa, there should be four inches between the front of the seat and the back of your knees. If you do not have this space, your lower back will be forced into a slouch, which strains your back and neck.

A good example of a chair with a seat cushion that is too deep is the recliner. The excessive seat depth (i.e., from front to back) of a recliner forces your lower back to slouch. The deep seats of a typical recliner only fit individuals who are over six feet four inches. If you are shorter than this, do not sit in standard-size recliners.

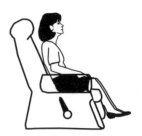

**Recliner Chairs
Cause Slouching**

If your chair or sofa seat is too deep, place an adjustable lumbar support [700] or a cushion behind your back. This support should be thick enough to move you forward on the sofa or chair so that the back of your knees are three to four inches in front of the edge of the seat cushion.

The height of the seat is also important. If the seat is too low, your legs will be forced straight out in front of you. This posture pulls on your lower back, rounding it, and simultaneously causes your neck to bend forward, stretching your ligaments, muscles, and nerves. In addition, your chair and sofa seat should be high enough to allow you to get in and out easily without straining your back or neck.

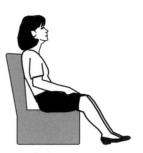

**Too-Low Chair
Causes Slouching**

If the seat of your chair or sofa is too low, place an additional cushion beneath your seat cushion to raise the seat height. Raising your chair or sofa seat to the proper height allows your lower back to rest against the lumbar support of the seatback, relaxing your lower back muscles, automatically allowing your neck muscles to relax too.

When a chair or sofa seat is too high, your feet

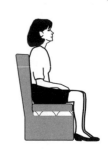

**Add Cushion
to Low Chair**

will not rest flat on the floor. The pressure of the seat on the back of your thighs will cut off the circulation of your legs as well as force you to lean forward, stretching the ligaments and muscles of your neck. If your seat is

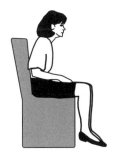

**Too-High Chair Causes
Rounded Posture**

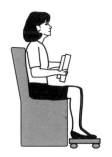

Place Feet on Footrest

too high, place a footrest under your feet to raise your knees. The footrest should be high enough to raise your knees slightly higher than your hip joints. The footrest should be stable and not shift around when used.

When the back of a chair or sofa seat is significantly lower than the front edge, it creates pressure on the back of the thighs and this cuts off the circulation to your lower legs. If the back of a chair or sofa seat is too low, add a wedge-shaped pillow [701] to raise yourself to the proper height.

THE CHAIR OR SOFA BACK

The back of your chair or sofa should be firm, angled fifteen degrees backward, and have a good lumbar (lower back) support. The posture this creates allows your back and neck muscles to relax.

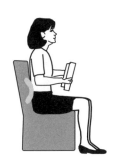

There should be a space at the bottom of the chair or sofa back for your buttocks, actually allowing your buttocks to protrude beneath it. If your chair or sofa does not have space for your buttocks, it will push your buttocks forward, forcing your lower back into a slumped position, which will cause your neck to slump forward.

**Chairs Should Have
Lumbar Support**

To correct this problem in a chair or sofa that does not have space for your buttocks, add a high-quality adjustable lumbar support [700] behind you. A properly adjusted lumbar support places your lower back into a forward curve. And, when you have a normal forward curve in your lower back, you will automatically have a tendency to have a normal forward curve in your neck.

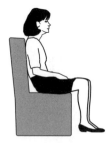 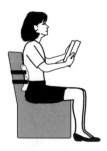

Lack of Space for Buttocks Causes Rounded Posture

Add Lumbar Support to Correct Posture

When using a lumbar support, position it so that it fits into the small of your back at the height of your belly button, not under your buttocks. Your body should be able to sink into the lumbar support with your buttocks protruding slightly backward beneath it. Be careful not to allow your buttocks to be pushed forward by a lumbar support that is positioned too low, as this will force your lower back and neck into a slumped position, causing a neck strain.

Your chair and sofa back should be high enough to support your lower and mid back. The upper part of the chair or sofa back should not be so thick that it forces your neck forward. If your chair or sofa has a thick roll at the top, use an additional cushion in the middle of the chair back to avoid pushing your neck forward.

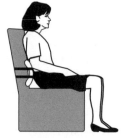 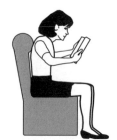 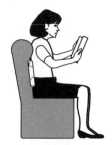

Too-Low Placement of Lumbar Support

Chair Roll Causes Bent-Forward Posture

Add Cushion to Chair

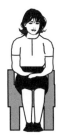 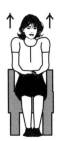 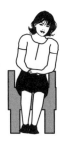

Correct Height   **Armrests Too High**   **Armrests Too Low**
of Armrests

ARMRESTS

The armrests of your chair or sofa should be padded and high enough for your elbows to rest comfortably on them, and they should extend to the front of the seat. When your arms rest at the proper height, the muscles of your neck and shoulders are able to relax. If the armrests are too high, they will push your shoulders up, bunching up your shoulder muscles, causing tension. If the armrests are too low, they will not give your arms the necessary support and you will have to bend your entire body to one side or crouch forward to rest your elbows on them. Remember, each arm weighs more than a bowling ball. When the weight of your arms pulls downward on your neck and shoulder muscles, these muscles can become strained.

If your chair or sofa has armrests that are too low, place pillows on them to raise them to the proper level. If your chair or sofa does not have armrests, place enough pillows on either side of you to make

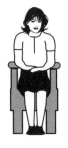 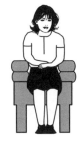 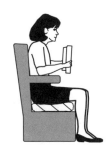

Add Pillows   **Create Armrests**   **Raise Body Height**
to Armrests   **with Pillows**   **with Pillow**

armrests of adequate height from them. Then rest your arms on the pillows. If your armrests are too high, add an additional seat cushion to raise your body high enough that your elbows and forearms rest correctly on the armrests.

SWIVEL

The ideal chair can swivel. Turning your entire body as one unit is far less strenuous on your neck than is twisting just your neck.

READING LAMPS

If you like to read, you owe it to yourself to have a good reading light. Unfortunately, most people make do with inadequate, dim lighting from a decorative lamp. Most ceiling or decorative lamps provide ambient lighting for lighting a room, which is good for being able to locate items but is horrible for reading.

Each reading area of your home should have an individual adjustable narrow-beam reading light [472]. This type of lamp should have a small, well-shaded head that is flexible and cool to the touch that will illuminate an area wide enough for a large book. These types of lights are available in table and floor models. Do not purchase lamps that are difficult to adjust, that do not stay in the adjusted position, that resist you when you are adjusting them, or that spring back to a preset position. Your constant attempts to reset these lamps to your reading needs will produce stress to your neck and arms.

READING TABLES AND MAGNIFIERS

Excellent additions to your reading areas are tilted reading tables and adjustable reading magnifying devices.

Think about your reading posture: hours go by with your head and neck bent forward and downward. This motionless activity, with your head and neck unsupported, places a tremendous strain on your neck and shoulder muscles and ligaments. Most of this strain can be eliminated by moving your reading material upward. The less you have to bend your head forward and downward, the less you will strain your neck. The solution is placing your reading material on an adjustable tilted reading table [473]. These tables come in many sizes and varieties. Some even have drink holders and bookshelves.

If you have trouble reading smaller print and have to bend your head closer to your reading material, you will strain your neck muscles. An adjustable reading magnifying device [474] will help you maintain correct posture while reading.

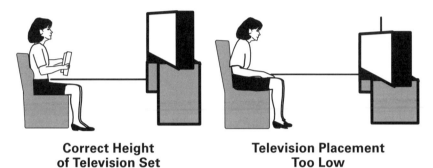

**Correct Height
of Television Set**

**Television Placement
Too Low**

The TV Set

Nowadays, people spend a great deal of time in front of the television. That is why it is so important to have correct posture when doing so. Practice the following TV placement guidelines to keep your neck healthy.

Place your TV at eye level, and always sit up to watch it. Generally speaking, make sure your TV screen is at least two to three feet off of the floor to prevent bending your head and neck forward or downward to watch it. Similarly, avoid placing your TV screen above three feet from the floor, or you will have to bend your neck backward and upward to view the screen. This can also happen if a large screen is placed too close to you. Prolonged viewing with your head and neck in this latter position strains your neck muscles, compresses the facets, and irritates the nerves of your neck.

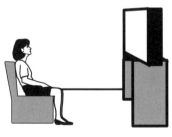

**Television Placement
Too High**

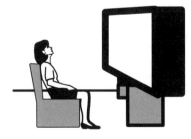

**Sitting Too Close to
Large Television Screen**

Children's Furniture

As we have discussed, furniture is not one-size-fits-all and unfortunately most furniture does not adjust to fit our bodies—our bodies must adjust to fit it. So, you can imagine what your body would go through if you were a three-foot-tall child forced to sit for any length of time in a chair designed to accommodate a six-foot-tall adult. Furniture that is either too big or too small for a child forces the child to sit with his or her back rounded, which causes his or her neck to slump forward. Over time, this creates a habit of bad posture and strains the muscles of the child's back and neck continuously.

To assist with the development of good posture, a child needs furniture that fits his or her individual size; therefore, the furniture needs to be adjustable or replaced to fit the child as he or she grows.

You can tell if the chairs your children sit in are too big for them when they slump while using a table, sit on their hands, sit with their knees up, support themselves on their elbows, or have trouble writing neatly. Adjustable chairs for children should have two essential features: an adjustable seat and an adjustable footrest. Do not purchase a chair in which only the seat is adjustable because as the seat is adjusted upward, the child's feet are left dangling, placing pressure on the blood vessels at the back of their thighs.

Furniture of particular importance nowadays is a child's computer work or play station. Many children love to play electronic games and to play on the computer. They can spend hours at a time there. As a result, one of today's most common causes of poor posture is a computer work or play station that does not fit the size of the child, forcing the child into an improper posture. So, for your child's health, always follow this rule: Continuously increase the size of your child's furniture as he or she grows, especially his or her computer desk and chair.

Parents can purchase an adjustable computer work or play station [475] that is easily adjusted to fit their child's growing height. Also, please refer to Chapter 14 to learn how to modify a computer desk and chair to fit anyone's size.

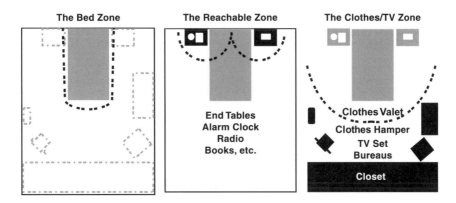

Bedroom Zones

Neck-Proofing Your Bedroom

The ergonomically correct, and easier-to-use, bedroom is composed of three zones: the bed zone, the reachable zone, and the clothes/TV zone. If you will organize your bedroom according to these zones, you will reduce the amount of reaching, stretching, and straining you will have to do each day.

THE BED ZONE

Placed in this zone are: the correct bed for your body (as described in Chapter 4), an ergonomically correct cervical pillow, an adjustable bed back support (Bed Lounger) [401], and a reading pillow [402] or tilting bed tray [403]. Multiple throw pillows, while pretty, require a lot of reaching and stretching to place them and take them off the bed … a lot of unnecessary work that can add strain to your neck. Tilting bed trays or, preferably reading pillows reduce the amount of forward bending you will have to do to read, which reduces the strain to your neck and frees your hand and arm muscles from holding your book in place.

THE REACHABLE ZONE

This zone contains everything you must be able to reach while in bed, such as an adjustable reading lamp, television remote controls, alarm clock, radio, books, etc. All of these items should be placed within easy reach on the nightstand alongside the bed. Personal items, such as medication, would be placed in the drawers of the nightstand.

THE CLOTHES/TV ZONE

This zone contains your bureaus, clothes valet, clothes hamper, TV, and closet. A clothes valet takes up little space and provides a handy place to hang your clothes until you find the time to put them in your closet, thereby reducing a lot of bending, lifting, stooping, etc.

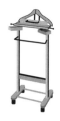

Clothes Valet

THE CLOSET

Compartmentalize your closet into separate areas for shoes, skirts and pants, shirts and blouses, suits and dresses, sweaters, and other garments. An ergonomically arranged closet eliminates dead space, makes it easier for you to find your clothes, and protects your neck.

Hats		Seldom used items	
Sweaters		Seldom used items	
Frequently Used Shirts, Blouses and Skirts	Pants and Dresses	Suits	Frequently Used Coats
Seldom Used Shirts, Blouses and Skirts			Seldom Used Coats

Correct "Body to Closet Storage" Relationship

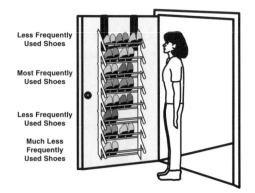

Less Frequently Used Shoes

Most Frequently Used Shoes

Less Frequently Used Shoes

Much Less Frequently Used Shoes

Correct "Body to Shoe Storage" Relationship

Arrange your closet so that all of your frequently worn clothes are hung at eye to elbow height. Place your shoes in a hanging shoe bag or rack [477] attached to the back of the closet door. The most frequently worn shoes should be placed between elbow and shoulder height. Place the shoes you wear the least at the bottom of the shoe bag or rack.

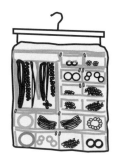

**Hanging
Jewelry Organizer**

Instead of fumbling, bending over, and reaching to find a piece of costume jewelry, hang your jewelry in your closet on a hanging jewelry organizer [478]. By placing your jewelry between eye and chest level, you will reduce the strain you place on your neck.

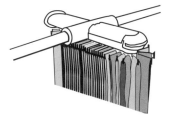

Motorized Tie Organizer

The same principle applies to reaching for men's ties. A motorized tie organizer [479] that hangs in a closet will reduce the bending, stretching, and stooping usually accompanying this task. The less bending and stooping you have to do, the less strain will occur to your neck.

Neck-Proofing Your Bathroom

BATHROOM VANITIES

The ideal height of a bathroom vanity is at waist level. If your vanity surface is too low, and it is not possible to permanently raise it, raise it by placing a small suitcase, an upside-down drawer, a thick kitchen chopping block, or an additional over-the-sink shelf [464] on the vanity surface. Then place your toiletry articles on these higher levels. Raising your vanity surface in this manner will reduce the forward bending of your head and neck when reaching for your toiletries.

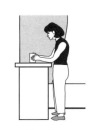

**Correct "Body to Vanity"
Surface Relationship**

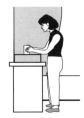

Raising Vanity Surface

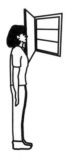
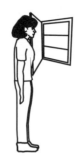
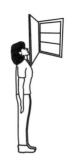

Correct "Body to Medicine Cabinet" Relationship

Medicine Cabinet Too Low

Medicine Cabinet Too High

MEDICINE CABINETS

Place your most frequently used toiletry articles, medicines, and vitamins between shoulder and eye height to avoid looking down or up for them. Looking downward stretches the muscles, joints, and discs of your neck, and looking upward jams the bony structures at the back of your neck.

BATHROOM MIRRORS

People often bend over to shave or apply makeup, which strains the muscles of the neck and back. To avoid this bending, you need an adjustable mirror[480] that is separate from your medicine cabinet or stationary bathroom mirror. This separate mirror can be mounted on a wall, as long as it can be pulled toward you. Another option is to purchase a mirror that is on a stand[481]. By placing this standing mirror close to you, you will be able to shave and apply makeup without bending your neck.

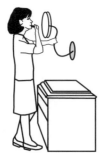
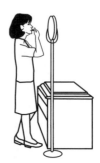

Adjustable Mirror

Mirror on a Stand

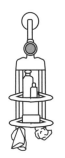

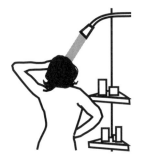

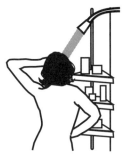

**Add-On
Shower Shelves**

**Add-On Triangular
Shower Shelves**

**Shower Shelves
on Pole**

YOUR SHOWER

As discussed in Chapter 6, in the shower it is important to reduce the amount of bending you do when reaching for soap, shampoo, sponges, and so on. One solution is to add shower shelves by attaching them to your showerhead [454], by adding triangular shower shelves [453] in the corner of your shower, or by placing shower shelves on a pole [455] in the corner of your shower. Place these new shower shelves so that the main shelf is between the height of your elbow and shoulder to prevent bending your head and neck forward to look or reach for items.

Replace your showerhead and controls with a sliding showerhead that can be adjusted upward to fit the tallest member of your family and downward for your children. These showerheads can change the shower height, spray intensity, and direction to match each family member's needs. In addition, it is wise to set your water heater's temperature low enough to avoid an accidental scalding.

Another great shower tip is to use a hose attachment [482] on your showerhead to rinse the

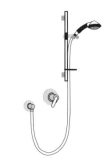

Sliding Shower Head

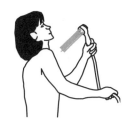

Use Hose Attachment

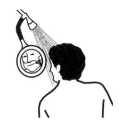

Use Fog-Free Mirror

soap from your body or the shampoo from your hair. You will still need to be conscious of not bending or straining your neck when doing these activities. Also, gentlemen, you can add a fog-free mirror [450] to your shower to shave without having to bend your neck forward.

BATHTUB

If you have to struggle getting in or out of a bathtub, consider replacing your existing tub with a walk-in bathtub [483]. All strains and sprains caused by entering and exiting a bathtub are eliminated with this type.

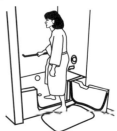

Walk-In Bathtub

TOILET PAPER HOLDERS

Also touched upon in Chapter 6, something as minor as reaching around behind you for toilet paper can cause a strain to your neck muscles. Toilet paper holders should be placed directly in front of you or at your side in front of you—never behind you. If your toilet paper holder is behind you, it will force you to twist your shoulders and neck to reach the paper, straining your neck. If your bathroom's toilet paper holder is not in the proper place, put your toilet paper on a small table in front of you, or get a free-standing toilet paper holder [463] and place it at your side in front of you.

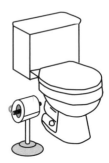

**Free-Standing
Toilet Paper Holder**

Neck-Proofing Your Pool Area

An outdoor reclining chaise lounge [484] is available that allows you to lie facedown without having to twist your head and neck to the side or stretch your head downward over the top of the chaise. This lounge allows you to comfortably read while laying facedown with absolutely no stress to your neck muscles.

Neck-Proofing Your Utility Room

WASHERS AND DRYERS

Almost all washers and dryers present an ergonomic nightmare. These appliances are built too low, with a door on top where you have to stretch up and over to be able to look down into the appliance, or with a door in front that requires you to bend over to about knee level to look inside. The havoc each of these bending and stretching maneuvers creates on your neck is made worse when you transfer handfuls of wet, heavy laundry from one appliance to the other. Thank goodness, washers and dryers built higher and with larger front doors at about hip to shoulder level were recently introduced to the market. These newly designed appliances will significantly reduce or eliminate the bent-forward or stooping postures that strain your neck and upper back.

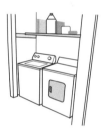

If you have the older, too-low washer and dryer, install a wall shelf over them. If your washer and dryer are the higher ones (as previously described), install a wall shelf at waist height to the side of them. The wall shelf is a place to store your detergents, water softeners, bleach, and so on. The bending and reaching for these items when placed in cabinets can be avoided when they are within easy reach.

Shelf Above Washer/Dryer

SEWING MACHINES

The height of a sewing machine work surface should be one and a half inches above your elbow height. If necessary, raise your sewing machine work surface to the proper height by placing wooden or plastic blocks[485] beneath it. Having your sewing machine at the right height for your body

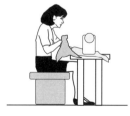

Correct Height of Sewing Machine

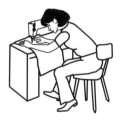

Straining Neck While Sewing

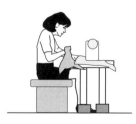

Add Blocks to Raise Sewing Machine

will reduce the repetitious bending of your head and neck forward and downward to sew.

IRONING BOARDS

Having your ironing board at the proper height will prevent your needing to lean over it. The height of an ironing board work surface should be one and a half inches above your elbow height. If your ironing board is too low, and not adjustable, raise it by placing it on a wooden box the length of the board (make sure the box has a non–slip surface to prevent accidents) or on wooden or thick plastic blocks.

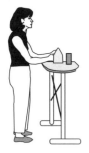
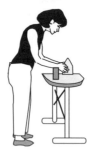
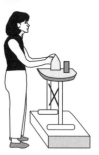

| **Correct "Ironing Board to Body" Relationship** | **Height of Ironing Board Too Low** | **Raise Ironing Board to Proper Height** |

The neck-aids and neck-appliances described in this chapter can be ordered through your family chiropractor or from the Neck and Back Products store at **www.NeckAndBackProducts.com** or call toll-free **1-800-882-4476.**

13

Neck-Proofing Your Vehicle

As discussed in Chapter 8, driving or riding in a vehicle can damage your neck. This happens in two main ways: 1) The improper postures and movements of your neck and body while in a vehicle can strain your neck muscles, and 2) excessive vibrations of a moving vehicle can damage your intervertebral discs, the cushions between your bones. Therefore, neck-proofing your vehicle is necessary to maintaining a pain-free neck. In this chapter, we will look at the different things you can do to make driving or riding in a vehicle more neck-friendly.

EXCESSIVE VIBRATIONS

Excessive vibrations from cars or trucks weaken the ligaments and discs in your neck and increase your chances of rupturing a disc and developing arthritis in your neck.

If you have a vehicle that produces too much vibration and cannot or do not want to purchase a more "neck-friendly" vehicle to reduce these vibrations, you can place specially designed vibration-dampening cushions[103] on your vehicle's seat. Other suggestions to lessen the harmful effects of a vehicle's vibration on your neck are: 1) avoid rough roads when possible, 2) reduce your speed when traveling over bumpy terrain, 3) keep your tire pressure correct, and 4) keep your vehicle's shocks, tires, and seat cushions in excellent condition.

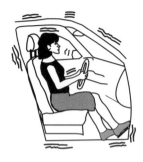

Excessive Vibrations

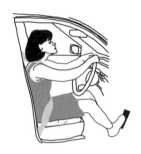

Vibration-Absorbing Pillow

ROAD JARRING

Jolts and jars produced by your vehicle that toss you around in your seat are called "road jarring." As noted in Chapter 8, some vehicles actually turn their occupants into human shock absorbers. To counter the ill effects of road jarring, make sure you tightly secure your seat belt whenever the vehicle is moving. To ensure the best protection, you also need to sit on a thick feather pillow or a vibration-dampening cushion, mentioned above. This thick pillow or cushion will help absorb some of the bouncing and jarring of the moving vehicle, thus making your body less of a shock absorber. Without this extra pillow or cushion, the vibrations and road jarring may injure the discs and ligaments of your neck and strain your neck muscles.

Neck-Proofing Your Vehicle's Seats

THE FIRMNESS OF YOUR VEHICLE'S SEAT

The ideal firmness of a vehicle seat is medium firm. If the seat is too soft, it will not hold your correct posture. Your body will slump, your neck will bend excessively forward, and, as you know, your neck muscles will be strained. You can tell that your vehicle's seat is too soft if your body indents the seat more than one inch. To correct a seat that is too soft, place a stiff plastic support seat [104] on your vehicle's seat to stiffen it.

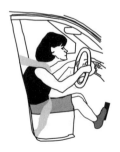

Vehicle Seat - Too Soft

If you must sit in a vehicle with seats that are too hard, simply place a feather pillow (not foam rubber), or a special liquid-filled pillow [105] on your seat. Sitting on these pillows will soften the effect of your vehicle's hard seat.

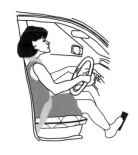

Liquid-Filled Pillow

THE DEPTH OF YOUR VEHICLE'S SEAT

If the seat of your vehicle is too deep from front to back, it will force your lower back into a back-ward curve, which will force your neck to bend forward, straining both structures. You can tell if your vehicle's seat is too deep if the front edge of the seat rubs the back of your knees. There should be three to four inches between the front of the seat and the back of your knees. If your seat is too deep, place an adjustable backrest (lumbar sup-port) [100] behind your lower back to give it the proper support.

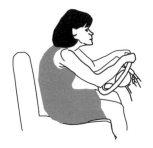

Too-Deep Car Seat Causes Poor Posture

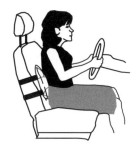

Adjustable Lumbar Support

THE HEIGHT OF YOUR VEHICLE'S SEAT

Your vehicle's seat should be high enough that with the bottoms of your feet comfortably on the floor, the position of your knees is about one inch above your hip joints, and the backs of your lower thighs are slightly above the front edge of the car seat. You should sit high enough to see easily and clearly over the steering wheel.

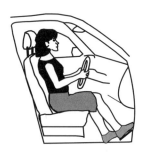

Correct Driving Posture

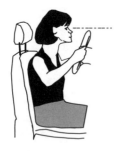

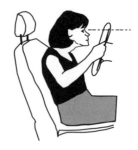

Car Seat - Too Low   **Car Seat - Too Low**

Sometimes people of short stature have to bend their head and neck downward to look under a steering wheel or crane their neck upward to look over a steering wheel. Both of these movements will produce a neck strain.

If you have to stretch your neck up and forward to see over the steering wheel, or down and forward to look under it, or if the front of the seat places pressure on the back of your thighs, you need to raise the height of your seat. If your seat cannot be automatically adjusted, place a car seat riser cushion [106] on the seat to raise yourself, or have a mechanic install wooden blocks under your seat to raise it to the proper height.

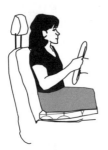

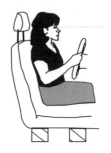

Car Riser Cushion   **Blocks Under Car Seat**

If the back edge of your car seat is significantly lower than the front edge, it will cause the front edge to press against the backs of your knees or lower thighs. This will restrict or cut off the blood flow to your lower legs. If the back edge of your car seat is too low, add a wedge shaped pillow [107] to raise yourself to the proper height.

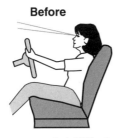 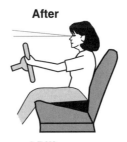

Before   **After**

Add Wedge-Shaped Pillow

THE SEATBACK

Your car's seatback should be firm, have a good lumbar (lower back) support, and be angled fifteen degrees backward. This configuration helps maintain your spinal curves, allowing your back and neck muscles to relax.

If your vehicle's seat does not recline fifteen degrees, attach an adjustable backrest (lumbar support) [100] to your seatback. The extra thickness of the lumbar support placed in your lower back at the level of your belly button allows your body to bend backward at the necessary angle. Buy an adjustable backrest that can be attached to the seat by a strap, to prevent it from sliding downward. If the lumbar support slides downward and is thus too low on your back, it will cause the strains you are trying to avoid.

When your vehicle's seat is leaning backward more than fifteen degrees, it forces your head to lean forward, pulling on your neck muscles, straining them. If your seat leans backward at too great an angle and cannot be adjusted to the proper position, place a wedged-shaped cushion [107] behind you with the thicker portion of the cushion at your shoulder level and the narrow portion near your buttocks, or use an add-on headrest [101].

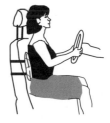

Adjustable Lumbar Support

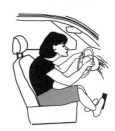

Seat Leaning Too Far Back

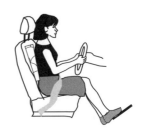

Add Wedge-Shaped Pillow

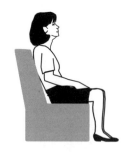

**No Space at
Bottom of Seatback**

There should be a space at the bottom of your seatback to allow your buttocks to protrude slightly beneath it. If your seatback does not have this feature, the seatback will push your buttocks forward, forcing your lower back to slump. As you know by now, this forces your neck to bend in the opposite direction, straining it.

If your vehicle's seat does not allow your buttocks to fit under the seatback, add a quality adjustable lumbar support to your vehicle's seatback by following the previously described directions.

CAUTION: Many commercially available lumbar supports are made of foam rubber and are too soft to provide adequate lumbar support. Be careful of the lumbar support you choose.

THE HEADREST

The top of the headrest should be positioned to be at the same height as the top of your head, and the entire headrest should be positioned within two inches of your head. In the event your vehicle's headrest is not sufficiently adjustable to accomplish these positions, attach an add-on headrest [101] to your vehicle to accomplish these tasks.

THE POSITION OF YOUR VEHICLE'S SEAT

In order for you to maintain good posture while driving, your vehicle's seat should be positioned so that the front of your body is exactly twelve inches from the steering wheel.

When a vehicle's seat forces your body to be closer than twelve inches from the steering wheel, you must awkwardly bend your arms to steer the vehicle. Every time you make a tight turn you will be placing increased muscle tension on your neck and shoulder muscles, straining them.

Likewise, if your seat is positioned too far back, you will have to stretch to grasp the steering wheel. This position will force you to bend your

**Seat Too Close
to Steering Wheel**

neck forward in order to drive, straining your neck muscles.

If you find yourself stretching to reach the gas and brake pedals, adjust your seat forward so you can place your heel on the floor and easily pivot the ball of your foot onto the gas and the brake pedals while maintaining your correct sitting posture. You should be able to use your vehicle's pedals by simply pivoting your foot, and not have to use your legs, hips, or back muscles.

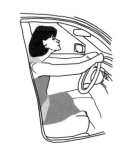

Seat Placed Too Far Back

If you cannot move your seat far enough forward to get in this position, place an adjustable lumbar support between your body and your vehicle's seatback. The support should be of sufficient thickness to place your body the proper twelve-inch distance from the steering wheel.

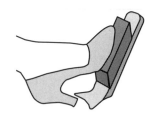

Add Blocks to Foot Pedal

If, after adjusting your vehicle's seat upward to place your body at the proper height and the seatback places your body the correct distance from the steering wheel, you find that your feet still do not reach the gas and brake pedals, have a mechanic add wooden blocks to these pedals to bring them closer to you. The mechanic should make sure the thickness of these blocks is sufficient to bring the surface of these pedals up to your foot. Ask your mechanic to place a non-slippery rubber surface on the blocks to keep your foot from slipping on them.

"Neck-Friendly" Adjustments to Your Rearview Mirrors

Your rearview mirrors should be adjusted so that you do not have to lean forward or twist your neck to use them. Position your side-view mirrors so that you only have to turn your head minimally to the right or left to view them. Also, tilt your rearview mirror slightly

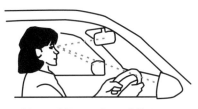

Use of Rearview Mirrors

upward. This will force you to maintain an upright sitting posture while driving.

Rotating your head to look over your shoulder when backing up a vehicle wrings your neck. Instead, try using your rearview and side-view mirrors to accomplish this task. If your vehicle does not have side-view mirrors, have a mechanic install them on both sides.

Another easy, neck-friendly side-view mirror modification is the addition of "fisheye"

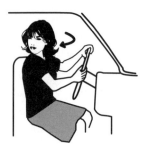

Don't Rotate Head to Look Over Shoulder

mirrors[108]. "Fisheye" mirrors are small convex mirrors that are applied to one lower corner of each of your existing side-view mirrors using a type of two-sided adhesive. "Fisheye" mirrors will eliminate your vehicle's "blind spots" (those spots that regular mirrors don't allow you to see), thereby eliminating the need for you to look over your shoulder, wringing your neck in order to see.

To improve side-view vision and decrease neck strain, you may also consider replacing your existing side-view mirrors with larger ones.

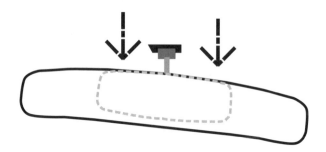

Panoramic Rearview Mirror

Special add-on panoramic rearview mirrors[109], while slightly distorting the images you are looking at, allow you to look out your back window and along both sides of your vehicle at the same time, thus reducing the necessity of twisting your neck to see what is going on around you.

Remember, the more you can see with your vehicle's mirrors, the less you will have to look over your shoulder and twist your neck.

The Proper Placement of Your Vehicle's Armrest

Using armrests while driving or riding in a vehicle will reduce the fatigue of your neck and shoulder muscles. Your armrests should be high enough to support your elbows and forearms without your having to lean forward or sideways to rest your forearms on them. Leaning to use an armrest creates stress on your neck.

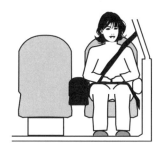

Correct Use of Armrests

If your vehicle's center armrest (between the two front seats) is too low, place a pillow on top of it to raise it to the proper height. And, if your vehicle does not have a center armrest, purchase a commercially available automotive armrest/console [110] and add it to your vehicle. If your window sills are too low to use as an armrest, add a padded armrest [111].

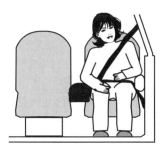

**Armrest
Too Low**

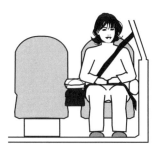

**Add Pillow
to Armrest**

Seat Belts

If the shoulder strap of your seat belt chafes your neck or uncomfortably compresses your breasts, add a "seat belt adjuster" [112] to it. The seat belt adjuster positions the shoulder strap several inches to the side, eliminating the chafing and reducing the pressure on your breasts.

Ease of Getting in or out of Vehicles

Getting into tall vehicles is often an awkward, straining event. Grabbing support handles to pull yourself upward places a strain on your neck, shoulder, and back muscles. Getting out of tall vehicles is equally awkward. And, crawling into and out of low vehicles also forces your body into contortions. An additional support handle [486] installed on the door, will assist you in getting in and out of vehicles that are too low or too high.

The neck-aids and neck-appliances described in this chapter can be ordered through your family chiropractor or from the Neck and Back Products store at **www.NeckAndBackProducts.com** or call toll-free **1-800-882-4476.**

14

Neck-Proofing Your Workplace When You Have a Sitting Occupation

The intent of this chapter is to help you develop an ergonomically perfect workplace. In today's modern office, the majority of a worker's activities are centered on his or her desk and chair. Workers sit for hours with their shoulders rounded, heads held forward toward their computer monitors, stressing their neck muscles. Therefore, proper ergonomics revolving around the sitting posture is extremely important.

Few work chairs or desk surfaces are designed to fit the human body. In fact, people are usually an afterthought when engineers design work furniture. The good news is that simple changes to an office workstation can create an optimal work site that alleviates existing strains and sprains and that prevents future problems.

Correct Sitting Posture

In order to reduce a repetitive strain injury of your neck at work, you will need to maintain correct sitting posture at all times. By placing your body in an optimal sitting posture, you will reduce or eliminate strains to your spine as well as the rest of your body. You will remember from Chapter 2 that correct sitting posture is when:

- You are sitting up straight, or leaning slightly backward without bending your neck.

- You are facing straight forward with your eyes straight ahead.

- The objects you are looking at are clearly visible by looking straight ahead or by simply tilting your eyes up or down.

- Your ear hole, mid shoulder, and hip are in a straight vertical line, or a line that leans slightly backward at the top, when viewed from the side.

- Your shoulders are resting comfortably on top of your rib cage.

- Your upper arms are hanging straight down.

- Your lower arms are bent at right angles to your upper arms, parallel to the floor, or preferably with your wrists slightly lower than your elbows, between ninety and one hundred degrees, with your forearms supported on the armrests. This position will allow your neck and shoulders to relax. However, if your hands and wrists are too low, your forearm muscles will tire.

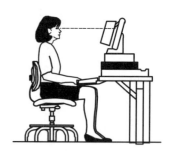

Correct Sitting Posture

- Your lower back is slightly arched forward and supported by the back of the chair.

- You are sitting all the way back in your chair with your buttocks against the back of the chair, not on the front edge.

- Your knees are slightly higher than your hip joints.

- The back of your lower thighs should be one inch above the front edge of your chair seat.

- Your calves should be at a right angle to your thighs, or preferably at slightly more than a right angle, between ninety and one hundred degrees, to reduce the pressure on the structures at the back of your knees.

- Your feet are flat on the floor or on a slightly elevated footrest.
- Your neck, shoulders, arms, and lower back are relaxed.

Sitting Work Neck Rules

SITTING WORK NECK RULE #1:
Keep your neck as still as possible; do not quickly bend your neck upward or downward, or turn it.
A sudden bending or turning of your neck can injure your neck muscles and spinal joints.

SITTING WORK NECK RULE #2:
Always face your work.
It is best to keep your neck in its normal, straight-ahead posture. Therefore, you need to face your work at all times. Keeping your neck in a turned position will quickly strain your neck muscles.

SITTING WORK NECK RULE #3:
While maintaining correct posture and without bending your neck, look straight ahead or simply raise or lower your eyes to view the objects you need to. Your goal should be to keep your head directly over your spine.

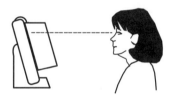

Look Straight Ahead

SITTING WORK NECK RULE #4:
Your desktop should be one and a half inches above your elbows when you are seated.

SITTING WORK NECK RULE #5:
Do not slump or slouch.
Slumping or slouching reverses the normal curve of your lower back, automatically causing the same reaction in the posture of your neck, straining it.

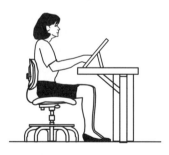

Correct "Work Surface to Body" Relationship

SITTING WORK NECK RULE #6:
Avoid bending your neck forward or leaning it to the side for long periods of time.

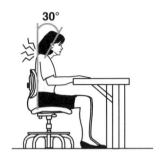

**Thirty-Degree
Bending of Neck**

The foremost rule for doing sit down work is to avoid constantly bending your neck forward and downward to see your work; for example, avoid bending over files for extended periods of time.

Try to maintain no more than thirty degrees of forward bending of your neck while reading, typing, or writing. A bent-forward posture, when maintained for a long period of time, can cause an overuse strain of your neck muscles.

Avoid leaning your head to the side (as in cradling a telephone between your head and shoulders) or bending your neck in any direction for long periods of time, because these positions will cause your muscles to tighten. When one neck muscle becomes tightened or begins to hurt,

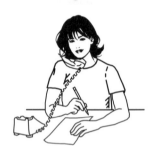

**Cradling Telephone
Causes Neck Strain**

its neighboring muscles also tighten up to help support the weight of your head. Prolonged tightened muscles produce a strain injury.

Also avoid rotating your head and neck for any length of time.

SITTING WORK NECK RULE #7:
Alternate the direction your neck is bending.

If your occupation forces you to hold your neck in one position for a prolonged period of time (e.g., bending, leaning, etc.), alternate the direction of the bend in your neck every ten minutes.

SITTING WORK NECK RULE #8:
Minimize overstretching to reach for work objects.

Whenever you overstretch to reach for objects, your arm muscles will pull on your neck, causing a strain to it.

Avoid Overstretching

SITTING WORK NECK RULE #9:
Take frequent stretch breaks.
Be sure to take a brief rest from your work every hour. Sitting in one position for long periods of time restricts the blood flow to these muscles, placing a tremendous amount of stress on your neck and shoulder muscles. To counter this muscle damage, get up and move around once every hour and go through three or four range-of-motion exercises (see Chapter 16). These exercises will increase the circulation to your muscles, relaxing them. The exercises will also return the circulation to the discs of your neck, helping prevent a disc injury.

Your Work Desk

The objective of ergonomics is to optimize the fit of the work environment (i.e., tools, work heights, etc.) to the individual worker. For example, the average height of a desktop is twenty-eight to twenty-nine inches. However, the correct height of a desktop is one and a half inches above the elbows of the person who is using it. Therefore, a tall person would need a taller desktop than someone shorter.

An ergonomically correct work desk [504] or adjustable computer desk [475] can be raised, lowered, and tilted; is large enough to hold all work items; and has ample space for your legs, two levels of work surfaces, a writing surface, and a keyboard surface.

As a side note, it is also wise to use a desk with a desktop that has rounded corners, in order to avoid injury when bumping into it.

THE HEIGHT OF YOUR DESKTOP

The ideal height of your desktop is one and a half inches above your elbows. This is low enough to prevent you from slouching forward and high enough to allow you to lean on the desktop. Resting your elbows on the desk when you are tired reduces the strain on your shoulders, upper body, and neck. This desktop height also allows your knees to slide easily under

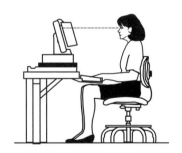

Correct
"Body to Work Desk"
Relationship

the desk, thus allowing your abdomen to come to the front of the desk.

If you work at a desk that is too low, you will tend to lean your head and neck forward and downward for long periods of time to bring your work closer to your eyes. This bent-forward position strains your neck muscles and hangs your head and neck on your ligaments, spraining them. This is one of the most common causes of neck pain. If your desktop is too low and not adjustable, build a box that is the same width and depth as your desk and that is tall enough to raise your work surface to the proper level. You may also place books or elevating blocks beneath the legs of your desk or place a large, thick chopping block on your desktop to lift your work surface to the proper height.

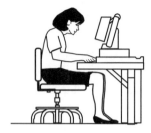

Desktop - Too Low

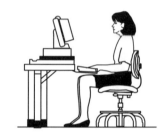

Elevating Blocks Under Desk

If your desktop is too high, you will hunch your shoulders upward to do your work, straining your upper back and neck muscles. If you cannot lower your desktop, sit in a chair that raises your body to match the ideal sitting posture.

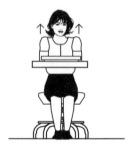

Desktop - Too High

The Angle of Your Desktop

If your work primarily consists of reading, consider inclining your desktop ten to fifteen degrees; that is, tilt it so that it is higher at the back than at the front. An inclined desktop reduces the need to bend your neck forward and to round your shoulders.

If you would like to incline your desktop and it cannot be tilted, place a larger slantboard [505] on your desktop surface with the front of it ten to fifteen degrees lower than the back. Place the new, angled surface on top

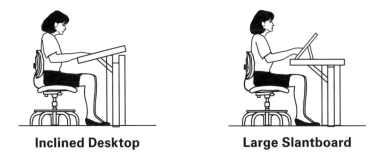

Inclined Desktop   **Large Slantboard**

of your old desktop. If your desk is large, place multiple slantboards on the desktop surface.

STORING MATERIALS

To increase the storage space for frequently used items, put them on a desk shelf[506] placed on the back portion of your desktop. These add-on shelves also free up your desktop for other materials.

Store frequently used and lighter items between elbow and shoulder height to minimize overhead reaching or bending to get into lower drawers or shelves. Store rarely used items in your lower desk drawers, with extremely heavy items at floor level on a dolly with wheels.

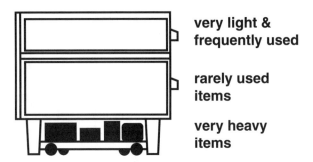

very light & frequently used

rarely used items

very heavy items

Storage of Items in Desk

Your Work Chair

Sitting in most work chairs is hazardous to your health. Poorly designed work chairs force you to sit in an awkward posture, causing injuries to your neck over time. The more time you spend sitting in poor posture, the more neck problems you will have. Without changing your posture, these problems will get progressively worse. The solution is to sit only in chairs that are uniquely designed to fit and support *your* neck and back.

Get in the habit of adjusting every chair you sit in as soon as you get in it. If, for example, you sit in a different work chair each day, you will need to start every workday by adjusting your chair. If you use the same work chair every day and it has been adjusted to fit you, you will not have to readjust it. However, whenever anyone else uses your work chair and changes its settings, you will need to readjust it to fit you each time you use it. This is like readjusting your car seat and rearview mirrors after someone else has driven your car.

ERGONOMICALLY DESIGNED WORK CHAIRS
Ergonomically adjustable chairs[507] are the best type of work chair, although usually somewhat expensive. However, they are not as expensive as the neck problems a poorly designed chair will create! An ergonomically designed work chair has many adjustable features to make your chair fit your height, size, and contours of your body for maximum support.

A properly fitted ergonomic work chair is one of the best investments a worker or company can make.

THE SEAT OF YOUR WORK CHAIR
Your work chair's seat should be adjustable—moving upward and downward, forward and backward, and tilting.

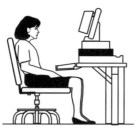

**Chair Seat
Too Long**

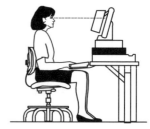

**Correct "Knee to Chair Seat"
Relationship**

The Front-to-Back Depth of Your Work Chair Seat
The depth of your work chair seat is important. The back of your knees should be four inches in front of the edge of the seat. This four-inch space prevents pressure from being put on the back of your calves and

therefore allows circulation to flow to your lower legs. A chair seat that is too deep from front to back will force your lower back to slouch, which will automatically cause your neck to slouch, straining your neck muscles and causing neck discomfort.

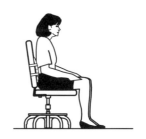

If your chair seat is positioned too far forward, slide it backward until you have the desired four-inch distance. If the seat is not adjustable, place an adjustable backrest (lum-

Adjustable Lumbar Support

bar support) [700] between your lower back and the back of your chair. The cushion should be thick enough to allow you to sit all the way back in the chair while having the proper space between the front of the seat and the back of your knees.

The Width of Your Work Chair Seat

Your work chair seat should be wide enough to allow your hips to move side-to-side.

The Height of Your Work Chair Seat

Your work chair seat needs to be high enough for you to get in and out of the chair easily, while still allowing you to place both feet comfortably and solidly on the floor. Your thighs should rest comfortably on the seat with your knees slightly higher than your hips and the front edge of the chair not digging into the muscles of your thighs.

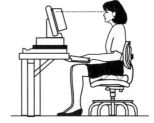

Add Cushion to Work Seat

If your work chair seat is too low and not adjustable, place a cushion on it. The cushion needs to be thick enough to raise you to the point that your knees are slightly above your hips.

If you adjust your chair height to attain the correct relationship to your desk height and find that you cannot place your feet comfortably on the floor or that the front of your chair seat puts pressure on the back of your thighs, you need to place your feet on a footrest [445]. Likewise, if your work chair seat is too high and not adjustable, you will need to use a footrest that is adjustable in height and incline (angle).

In cases like these, the footrest should be high enough to raise your knees to slightly higher than your hip joints. To make sure the footrest is stable enough to not move around when you are working, get one that is fourteen to eighteen inches deep and sixteen to twenty-four inches wide and with a non-skid surface.

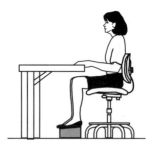

Add Footrest

If your chair seat is too high and crowds your knees under your desk, or positions your desktop too low in relationship to your body, raise your desktop. Do so by following the instructions in the "The Height of Your Desktop" section earlier in this chapter. Or, if it is impractical to raise your desktop, take the center drawer out of your desk to give yourself more legroom.

Tilting Your Work Chair Seat

Often, adjustable chairs will have the option of changing the tilt angle of the seat. The type of work you are doing will determine whether you need to tilt your chair seat upward or downward.

If you spend a great deal of time at work reading, writing, or otherwise bending over your desk, you will need to tilt the front of your work chair seat slightly downward. This drops the front of your thighs downward, which automatically puts a curve in your lower back, simultaneously creating the proper curve in your neck. However, a word of caution: Do not tilt the front of your work chair seat too far downward to the point that you feel like you are sliding off the chair.

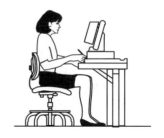

Lower Front of Chair Seat

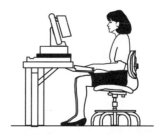

Raise Front of Chair Seat

If you operate a computer, are dictating, use a telephone a lot, or are in a meeting, you need to tilt the front of your seat upward five degrees. This will place your lower back against the lumbar support in your chair back, automatically guiding your neck into its proper posture. Do not, however, tilt the front of your seat upward more than five degrees because the front edge of the seat will dig into the back of your thighs, cutting off the circulation to your lower legs.

The Upholstery of Your Work Chair Seat

The seat of your work chair should be padded and have rounded front edges. The padding should not be soft; soft chair seats are for home use only. Rather, the seat of a work chair should be semi-firm. The seat's upholstery should not be too slippery in order to prevent you from sliding into a slouched position. At the same time, the seat should not be sticky or prevent free movement. The seat upholstery should be made of an absorbent material that breathes, such as cotton or leather.

THE BACK OF YOUR WORK CHAIR
Height

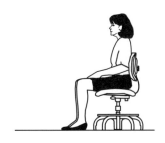

The back of your work chair should be high enough to support your lower and mid back and should be slightly wider than your torso. There should be a space for your buttocks between the bottom of the chair back and the top of the chair seat.

Correct Position of Seatback

Adjusting the Back of Your Chair Forward and Backward

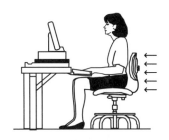

If your chair seat is not adjustable but the back of your chair is, and the seat is too deep from front to back, move the back of your chair forward until there is a four-inch space between the front of the chair seat and the back of your knees.

Similarly, if your chair seat is not adjustable and is not deep enough from front to back, move the back of your chair backward until you have a four-inch gap between the front of your chair seat and the back of your knees.

Adjusting the Seatback

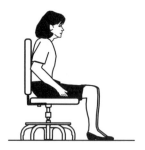
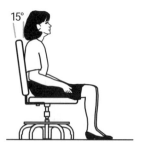

Lean Seatback Backward Fifteen Degrees

Tilt

As a general rule, the top of your work chair should be tilted backward ten to fifteen degrees. When you lean backward in this way, the stress on your spine is reduced, relaxing your neck and back muscles.

Lumbar Support

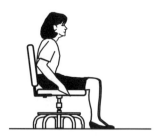

The position of your lower back in a work chair is extremely important because it influences the position of your neck. If the back of your chair does not have a lumbar support, your lower body will automatically slouch backward. This bends your neck forward, straining it. Therefore, always press your lower back against the lumbar support of the back of your chair in order to keep your neck in the proper position.

No Space for Buttocks

A properly placed lumbar support will support the natural curve of your lower back, holding it in a slightly arched position, and will also help

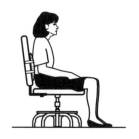

Add Lumbar Support

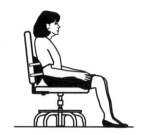

Lumbar Support Placement Too Low

support the weight of your upper body by diverting the weight of your upper back into the back cushion.

If your chair back does not have a lumbar support, use an adjustable backrest (lumbar support) [700] that can be attached by straps to the seat-back. Position this lumbar support in the curve of your lower back, at the level of your belly button. Placing it lower will push your buttocks forward, bending your lower back backward and simultaneously rounding your neck forward, straining it.

Tension

The tension of your chair's back will need to be adjusted according to your size and weight. The ideal tension is medium firm. The heavier the person, the more tension he or she will require. For example, a 250-pound man will need more tension in his chair back to support his weight when he leans backward than would a 150-pound man. If your chair back is too loose, you will end up leaning too far back and having to bend your head and neck forward to work.

THE ARMRESTS OF YOUR WORK CHAIR

A primary cause of shoulder and neck pain is poor or incorrect arm posture. Correct arm posture at work can be achieved by using properly placed armrests.

Sitting in a chair that does not have armrests can cause several different problems. Remember, arms are heavy, weighing more than a gallon of milk each. Thus, without armrests, the weight of your arms places significant downward pull on your upper back and neck muscles, causing strains, spasms, and pain in these muscles, as well as headaches.

No Armrests

To properly match your chair's armrests to the size of your body, the armrests will need to be adjustable up and down, forward and backward, sideways, and out of the way.

The armrests should be padded to provide a comfortable resting place for your arms and forearms during breaks.

The Height of Your Armrests

Adjust the armrests of your chair to the height at which your upper arms hang straight down to the armrests, with your elbows lifted slightly to take the tension off of your neck and shoulder muscles, your forearms resting on the armrests, and your arms and shoulders relaxed. Your wrists and hands should be slightly lower than your elbows. In this position, the armrests support the weight of your arms, thus reducing the pull of your neck and shoulder muscles and allowing your upper back and neck muscles to relax.

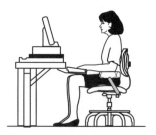

Correct Placement of Armrests

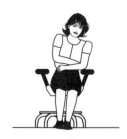

Armrests - Too Low

If your armrests are too low and are not adjustable, place pillows or cushions on them to raise them to the proper height. You know that your armrests are too low when you have to bend your whole body forward or to the side to reach them.

If your armrests are too high, they will push your shoulders upward, toward your ears, producing tension in your upper back and neck muscles and possibly pinching the nerves that go into your arms and hands. When your armrests are too high and are not adjustable, raise the seat of your chair until you sit high enough that your elbows are lifted slightly to take the tension off of your neck and shoulder muscles. Refer to the description of how to raise your chair seat found in the section "The Height of Your Work Chair Seat" earlier in this chapter.

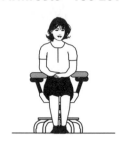

Add Cushions to Armrests

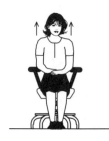

Armrests - Too High

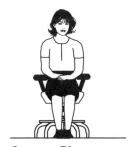
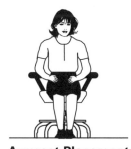
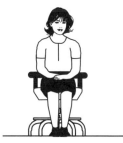

**Correct Placement
of Armrests**

**Armrest Placement
Too Far Apart**

**Armrest Placement
Too Close Together**

The Sideways Placement of Your Armrests

The best position for your armrests is directly under your elbows when your arms are hanging straight downward from your shoulders. When armrests are too far outward, a splayed elbow position strains your neck muscles. When armrests are too far inward, your elbows will repeatedly fall off of them, jerking on your neck muscles, straining them.

The Forward and Backward Placement of Your Armrests

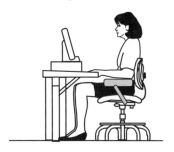

Computer users have a tendency to bring their shoulders forward in order to reach the keyboard, which strains the neck and shoulder muscles. Your armrests should be placed far enough backward to allow your chair to be close enough to your desk that your stomach can lean against the front of the desk. This position helps

**Correct "Armrests to
Work Surface" Relationship**

to prevent bending your head and neck forward while you work, straining your neck muscles.

THE SWIVEL FEATURE OF YOUR WORK CHAIR

Make sure your work chair can swivel (turn) so that you can easily face either side to reach for objects, such as manuals, books, and catalogs, or to reach into your desk's drawers. When possible, avoid turning or twisting your shoulders or neck to reach or look for anything. Twisting strains your neck. Instead, swivel your chair and entire body to look or reach in another direction.

If your chair does not have a swivel feature, you can place casters or rollers on your chair to rotate it. There are two types of casters available; choose the one most appropriate for your work area. Soft casters and rollers are best for hard surfaces, such as tile and linoleum floors. Hard casters and rollers are best for soft surfaces, such as carpets.

If your work chair sits on a carpet, place a Lucite or plastic mat under your chair to allow for easy movement. If you have to strain to move your chair, you may strain your neck muscles.

THE PROPER POSITION OF YOUR WORK CHAIR

Move your chair close to your desktop. Doing so will help prevent you from bending your head and neck forward and downward to view your work.

The Correct Placement of Objects on Your Work Surface or Desktop

The proper placement of materials and objects on your work surface or desktop is as important to the well-being of your neck as is maintaining proper posture. In fact, the two go hand in hand. To avoid straining your neck muscles, you need to lay out your work materials in such a manner that you can maintain normal posture at all times while using them. You should not have to overreach to grasp the materials you need. Improper placement of objects on a work surface or desktop will result in poor posture, the craning of your neck forward, your having to overstretch to reach for items, and the repetitious turning of your neck to look for objects.

Every worker needs to individually place the objects on his or her work surface or desktop to match the type of work he or she does. Reaching for objects poorly placed on a desktop or work surface will strain your neck muscles.

The following common sense guidelines will help you place objects properly on a sitting work surface or desktop. These also apply to standing work surfaces and to the desktops and surfaces you use at home, such as the kitchen counter.

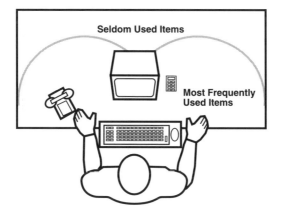

Placement of Items on Desktop

FREQUENTLY USED OBJECTS

To avoid straining your neck while sitting at your desk, place your most frequently used items directly in front of you within twenty inches of your body. This way you do not have to stretch to reach the objects and you reduce the number of times you turn your neck each day. Remember, minimizing the reaching distance and keeping your head and neck straight reduces your chances of neck strain.

Telephone

Place your telephone within twenty inches of your body on the side opposite your primary hand (i.e., the hand you use to write).

If your job requires you to use a telephone more than 20 percent of the day, get a hands-free headset[508], a speakerphone[501], or a built-up phone handle[509] to reduce the strain on your neck and to eliminate the headaches caused by cradling the phone between your head and shoulder. Headsets and speakerphones also free your hands to simultaneously conduct other work or home activities while using the telephone with your head and neck in a normal posture.

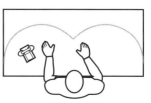

Placement of Telephone on Desktop

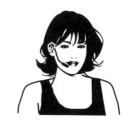

Hands-Free Headset

An articulating arm for telephones [510] allows you to pull a telephone up to you when in use and place it off your desktop when not in use, thus freeing up your work surface for other purposes.

Computer, Keyboard, and Monitor
The proper placement of these items is discussed at great length below.

Calculator
Place your calculator directly in front of the hand that will use it.

Hole-Punching Appliances
If you rarely use a hole-punching device, place yours outside the twenty-inch reaching distance. If you frequently use a hole-punching device, place the hole-puncher inside the twenty-inch reaching distance. As a side note, the pressure exerted to physically punch holes through a number of papers can strain your neck muscles. Ideally, it is best to use an electric hole-puncher to punch holes.

OBJECT PLACEMENT FOR SPECIFIC WORK SITUATIONS
If You Primarily Do Paperwork
If your job consists largely of doing paperwork, place your paperwork directly in front of you with your telephone in front of your non-primary hand. Place your computer monitor, keyboard, and mouse on the side of your primary hand, and your calculator to the side of the hand that will use it.

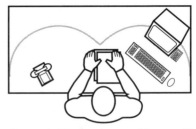

Correct Placement of Items If You Primarily Do Paperwork

If You Primarily Use a Computer
If your work is mostly using a computer, place your computer monitor directly in front of you and your keyboard on a keyboard tray [511] below the writing surface and slightly below elbow level. Place your mouse

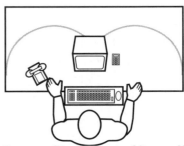

Correct Placement of Items If You Primarily Use a Computer

the same distance away from your body as the keyboard, next to your keyboard, with your telephone in front of your non-primary hand, and your calculator in front of the hand that will use it. This placement will reduce the number of times you have to turn your neck while working.

If You Primarily Do Paperwork and Do Not Use a Computer

Place your paperwork directly in front of you with your telephone in front of your non-primary hand and your calculator in front of the hand that will use it.

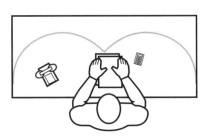

Correct Placement of Items If You Only Do Paperwork

If You Use a Telephone and Calculator Equally, and Do Paperwork

If your job requires you to use a telephone and calculator equally, and requires you to do paperwork, the following placement of materials will prevent you from repeatedly rotating your head and neck. Place your telephone in front of your non-primary hand, your paperwork directly in front of you, and your calculator to the side of the hand that will use it.

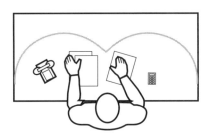

Correct Placement of Items If You Primarily Use Telephone, Calculator, and Paperwork

If You Primarily Use a Computer While Looking at Reference Materials

Place your telephone in front of your non-primary hand, your calculator in front of the hand that will use it, and your computer monitor directly in front of you with your keyboard and mouse on a keyboard tray [511] below the writing surface and slightly below elbow level. Place your reference

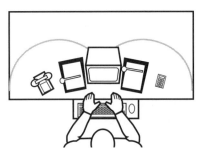

Correct Placement of Items If You Primarily Use a Computer and Reference Materials

materials in an upright document holder [512] located alongside your computer monitor on the side of your primary hand. Place an additional upright document holder on the opposite side of your monitor. To prevent turning your neck in only one direction, alternate the placement of your documents throughout the day. The document holders should be placed at slightly below eye level and closer to you than your computer monitor. Not using properly placed document holders is one of the most common causes of neck pain in computer operators.

If You Primarily Input Information from Written Materials and Rarely Look at Your Computer Screen

When the majority of your work consists of inputting into the computer from written material, it is most important to have the written source material in an upright document holder [512] or slant-board [503] directly in front of you. Your computer monitor is less often your visual focus, so it goes on the side of your primary hand. Place your keyboard and mouse in the keyboard tray under the writing surface at slightly below elbow

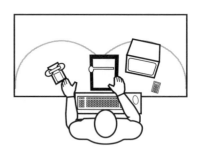

Correct Placement of Items If You Primarily Input Information and Rarely Look at Computer

level directly in front of you, your telephone in front of your non-primary hand, and your calculator in front of the hand that will use it.

Another option is to place your computer monitor on a moveable, "articulating" arm [513], which allows you to push the monitor further back when you are not looking at it and to pull it closer when you need to see the screen.

If You Primarily Type Information from Paperwork and Frequently Look at Your Computer Screen

Place your computer monitor directly in front of you with your keyboard and mouse on a keyboard tray below the writing surface at slightly below elbow level. Place upright document holders on either side of your computer monitor. Place the document holders closer to you than to your computer monitor to avoid having to bend your head and neck forward to read from them. To prevent turning your neck in only one direction, alternate the placement of your documents between the two document holders. Place your telephone in front of your non-primary hand and the calculator in front of the hand that will use it.

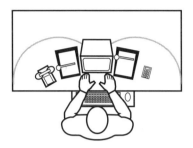

Correct Placement of Items If You Primarily Input Information and Frequently Look at Computer

Another option is to raise your computer monitor and place an extra-wide document holder[505] in front of it. This will prevent you from turning your head to refer to your paperwork.

Make sure all document holders are positioned so that you can look slightly downward with just your eyes to view the documents, rather than bending your head and neck downward. Better yet, rather than input-

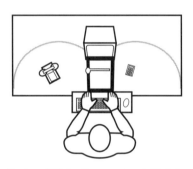

Extra-Wide Document Holder

ting, invest in a scanner to scan your documents into your computer.

If You Primarily Write Down Information from a Computer Monitor and Infrequently Input Information into Your Computer

Place your computer monitor directly in front of you with your writing materials in front of your computer monitor. Place your keyboard and mouse on a keyboard tray under the writing surface at slightly below elbow level. Also, place your telephone in front of your non-primary hand and the calculator in front of the hand that will use it.

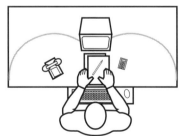

Correct Placement of Items If You Primarily Write Down Information from a Computer

If You Alternate Equally Between Looking at a Computer Screen and Paperwork to Be Typed

If you need to view both your computer screen and paperwork equally, place your computer monitor directly in front of you with your keyboard and mouse on a keyboard tray that is placed under the writing surface at slightly below elbow level. Place your paperwork in upright document holders attached to both sides of your computer monitor. To prevent turning your neck in only one direction, alternate the placement of the paperwork from one side to the other throughout the day. Place your telephone in front of the non-primary hand and the calculator in front of the hand that will use it.

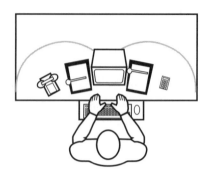

Correct Placement of Items If You Primarily Use a Computer and Reference Materials

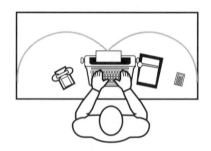

Correct Placement of Items If You Primarily Use a Typewriter and Look at Reference Material

If You Use a Typewriter (Not a Computer) and Input Information from Paperwork

Place your typewriter directly in front of you with your paperwork in a document holder on either side of your typewriter. Alternate the document holder from side to side throughout the day to reduce a one-sided strain. Place your telephone on the side of your non-primary hand and the calculator in front of the hand that will use it.

If You Use a Computer and Frequently Have to Refer to Heavy Catalogs or Books

Place your computer monitor directly in front of you, with your keyboard and mouse on a keyboard tray [511] that is placed below the writing surface at slightly below elbow level. Place your telephone in front of your non-primary hand and the calculator in front of the hand that will use it. To avoid straining your upper back and neck muscles, place your heavy books and catalogs on one side of your desk or on a desk return. The desk return should be placed at a right angle to your desk so that you can easily roll your chair up to it when using the books or catalogs.

As a note of caution, do not place heavy catalogs and reference books at a low level because you will strain your neck muscles when bending over to read from them or when reaching for and lifting them.

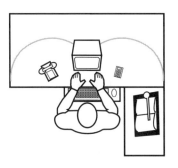

Correct Placement of Items If You Primarily Use a Computer and Refer to Heavy Catalogs/Books

SLANTBOARDS OR BOOKSTANDS

Place heavy reading materials on a slantboard[503] or bookstand[514]. Make sure the slantboard or bookstand is placed at slightly below eye level and closer to you than is your computer monitor, so that you can read from the materials without bending your neck forward or downward. Alternate the slantboard

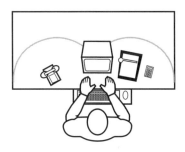

Use a Slantboard

or bookstand from one side of your computer monitor to the other throughout the day. If your slantboard is too low, raise it to the proper height by placing books beneath it.

Computer Monitors

Full-time computer operators who have ergonomically correct placement of their computer monitors and keyboards turn their necks approximately 3,000 times a day. An improperly placed computer monitor and keyboard will triple the number of times you will have to bend and rotate your neck in a day. And, as you know, the more you bend and twist your neck, the more you can injure it. Following is a discussion about the proper placement of your computer monitor as well as other features that need to be considered when trying to properly position the computer monitor to best fit your body.

THE CORRECT PLACEMENT OF A COMPUTER MONITOR

The normal neck is curved toward the front. Whenever you look downward, the curve of your neck straightens or reverses direction. If your neck stays in the straightened or reversed position for any length of time, it will produce neck, shoulder, and upper back pain. The primary way to minimize the bending of your head and neck downward when using a computer is to place your computer screen at the proper height and distance from your eyes.

DISTANCE OF THE MONITOR FROM YOUR EYES

Computer vision strain is a term that describes the eyestrain produced by a computer monitor placed too far away from the computer operator. The user has to strain his or her eyes to see the screen. Computer operators also have a tendency to push their head forward to view the screen. This posture strains the neck and upper back and leads to a head-forward posture.

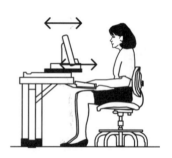

Setting Size of Letters on Computer

There are two steps in determining how far to place your computer monitor from your eyes to avoid having to lean forward to read the print. First, set the font size (size of the letters) and the zoom (size of the image on the screen) so that these are comfortable for you to read. Second, sit up straight and— keeping your neck straight—move your computer monitor toward and away from you until the letters are crystal clear. When the letters are crystal clear, your screen is the correct distance from your eyes.

THE HEIGHT OF YOUR COMPUTER MONITOR

The proper height of a computer monitor is with the top of the screen just slightly above eye level. If your computer monitor sits too far below your eye level, you will be forced to bend your head and neck forward and downward to read the screen. This posture, as you know, produces a neck strain. In fact, a primary cause of neck strain and pain in computer operators is a computer screen that is too low. We call this particular type of neck strain "computer neck."

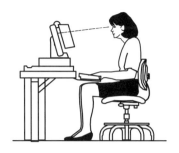

Position your computer monitor so you can see it without hanging your head down. You must be able to simply move your eyes to see all the words on your computer screen without moving your head or neck in any direction. As noted, constantly bending, leaning, or

Computer Screen Too Low

twisting to view your computer screen is one of the most common work-related causes of neck strain.

To adjust your computer monitor so that it is at the right height for you, first sit up straight with your head and neck in correct sitting posture. Then, raise the monitor until the top of the glass portion of your screen

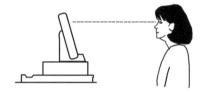

(not the plastic part) is slightly above your eye level. Another method of determining the proper height of a computer monitor is to place the middle of the computer screen at the level of your jaw. In this position, you will be able to keep your head and neck in a correct posture at all times while eas-

Correct "Eye to Computer Screen" Relationship

ily seeing the screen. This position will not strain your neck because you will not have to repeatedly bend your neck downward or upward.

If you have an oversized monitor, raise the monitor so that the top of the glass portion of the screen is four inches above your eye level. If your monitor's height is not adjustable, raise it to the proper height using the

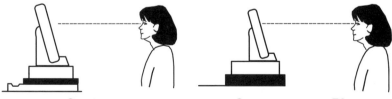

Correct "Eye to Oversized Computer Screen" Relationship

Computer on a Riser

right size "riser" [515]. You can, of course, also raise the monitor by placing it on top of a larger computer base, a box, or books. Larger computer bases can be purchased at a computer store.

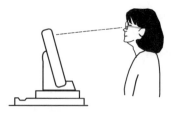

**Bifocals Cause
Head to Tilt Backward**

If you wear bifocal or trifocal glasses, you will need to place your computer screen slightly lower and closer to you than will people who do not wear these glasses. This is because the bottom lenses of bifocal or trifocal glasses are designed for reading words that are closer than those on a computer screen. When computer operators wear bifocal or trifocal glasses, they have to sit closer to the monitor and must continuously tilt their head upward to read the screen. This continuous tilting of the head up and down strains the neck muscles and contributes to headaches, neck pain, and a head–forward posture.

Therefore, if you wear one of these types of reading aids, first place your monitor in the correct position as described previously, then lower it one to two inches. This lower height prevents the need to tilt your head up to see the screen through your glasses. An even better solution would be to purchase single–vision glasses especially designed for computer use, those in which the entire lens magnifies the image equally.

If your computer monitor is too high for you and cannot be lowered, take the monitor off of its base (most have removable bases). Then, adjust the monitor to the right height by placing it on a lower computer base, on a riser, or on top of books.

Tilt

To further prevent bending your head and neck forward or downward, tilt the top of your computer monitor backward ten degrees so that the top of your computer screen is farther away from you than the bottom is. You should always look slightly downward when reading a monitor by

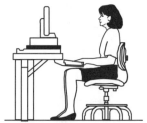

**Improper Tilt
of Computer Screen**

simply moving your eyes downward. If you think about it, we do not hold books directly in front of our eyes to read them, nor should we look directly at a computer screen when reading from it.

Glare

Glare on a computer screen is offensive to your eyes and will force you to constantly lift and lower your chin in an attempt to avoid

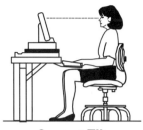

**Correct Tilt
of Computer Screen**

it. This repeated up-and-down motion strains your neck muscles. By tilting your computer monitor in the way described, you will reduce most or all of the glare that will appear on your computer screen. To further prevent glare, place your computer monitor at a right angle to any windows. Do not place the back of the monitor toward a window so that the computer screen is facing away from the window. Though this position would prevent the sunlight from hitting the screen, it would also put the sun in

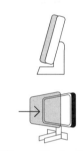

**"Glare-Reducing"
Screen**

your eyes, forcing you to constantly move your head to avoid it. Likewise, do not place the front of the computer monitor toward a window, as this position will pick up glare. If you have tried everything else and your computer screen still picks up glare, you can purchase a monitor that has a glare-reducing screen. A less expensive option would be to buy an anti-glare computer monitor hood [516] to shield your screen from glare.

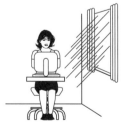

**Correct "Computer
Screen to Window"
Relationship**

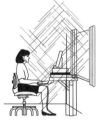

**Sunlight
in Your Eyes**

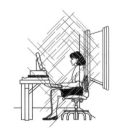

**Glare on
Computer Screen**

The best lighting for computer use is soft, indirect, or overhead lighting, because it produces minimal glare. Fluorescent lighting is fine as long as the light fixture is covered by a grid or shield. If you prefer not to use fluorescent lighting, purchase a special non-glare computer light [517].

Keep Your Computer Screen Clean

Having dust and fingerprints on a computer screen reduces the clarity of the words and images on the screen. A monthly cleaning will reduce your eyestrain.

ADDITIONAL FEATURES OF YOUR COMPUTER MONITOR

Size

If your computer screen is too small, you will have to bend your head and neck forward and downward to see it clearly. It is best to get a monitor with a screen that is at least fifteen to seventeen inches. The larger the monitor, the easier it will be to read.

Brightness

If your computer screen is too bright, it will strain your eyes when you try to read from it. You might not think this affects your neck, but it does—to avoid straining your eyes, you will automatically pull your head and neck backward to get away from the brightness. This backward bending of your neck places a strain on your neck muscles.

To determine what screen brightness is best for you, dim your computer screen until you have to strain to read it, then turn up the brightness until you reach a level that feels comfortable to your eyes.

Color Optimization

Use your color optimizer to select the color of the text (letters) and the background of your computer screen. A light background with clear dark letters is usually the easiest to read.

Articulating Arm

To create more workspace on your desk, you can add an articulating arm [513] to your computer monitor. This device allows you to easily

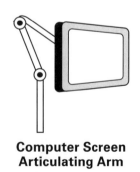

**Computer Screen
Articulating Arm**

move your monitor in front of you when you need to use it and then to just swing it out of the way when you do not need it.

Once you have your computer monitor correctly placed and adjusted to fit you, then ergonomically place the other objects you frequently use on your work surface or desktop.

Wall-Mounted Computer Monitor

If your desktop is small and your computer monitor takes up too much space, consider placing it on a wall mount [518]. A wall-mounted computer monitor allows you to pull the screen up to you when needed and push it out of the way when not in use.

Holding Your Paperwork

UPRIGHT DOCUMENT HOLDERS

As noted, upright document holders are important tools for anyone who needs to read paperwork while typing on a keyboard. If your occupation requires you to read a lot of documents, never place them flat on your desk. Placing your materials in a document holder or putting a book on a slantboard allows you to maintain normal posture. Document holders can be attached to either side of a standard computer monitor. In fact, it is a good idea to buy two of them and attach one to each side so that you do not need to move them when alternating sides. Another option is to purchase a document holder on an articulating arm [519], which allows you to pull the document holder into position when needed and push it out of the way when not in use.

To type from something you are reading, place your paperwork in one of the

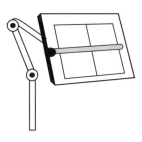

**Document Holder
Articulating Arm**

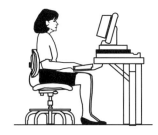

**Document Holder Attached
to Computer Screen**

upright document holders attached to your computer monitor. The document holders should be slightly below eye level and closer to you than the computer screen. To prevent the forward bending of your head and neck and to keep from constantly turning your neck to one side, alternate the placement of your paperwork from one document holder to the other.

If you do not have an upright document holder [512], utilize a free-standing clipboard or paper holder [520], placing it at the same height as your computer screen yet closer to your eyes, as explained above. Again, frequently move the clipboard or paper holder from one side to the other to prevent using only one side of your neck.

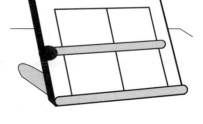

Desktop Document Holder

SLANTBOARDS AND BOOKSTANDS

As noted, if you need to type from reading materials that are too heavy to be placed in a document holder, such as books, large catalogs, and so on, use a slantboard [503] or bookstand [514]. Place the slantboard or bookstand slightly below eye level and closer to you than your computer monitor. Remember to

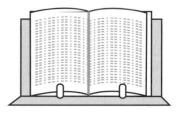

Slantboard/Bookstand

alternate the slantboard or bookstand from one side of your computer monitor to the other throughout the day. If your slantboard or bookstand is too low, raise it using books or another type of riser.

Scanner Placement

Because most people rarely use a scanner, this is usually best placed on the side of your non-primary hand and outside of the optimal reaching distance of twenty inches from your body. However, be sure to install your scanner so that it can be easily moved to the workspace directly in front of you when you need to use it. Better yet, if you have a return on your desk that is not needed for other more frequently used items, install your scanner there, thus eliminating the need to move it for usage.

Computer Keyboard

THE PLACEMENT OF YOUR KEYBOARD

As you know from reading this far, the ideal height of your keyboard is at slightly below elbow level. At this height, you do not have to strain your upper back or neck to use it, and you can see it without having to move your head.

Correct posture for using a keyboard is when your upper arms are hanging straight down; your forearms, wrists, and hands are slightly lower than your elbows; and your elbows are close to your body with the keyboard sitting just below your hand level. In this posture, your fingers will automatically be placed on the third row from the bottom of the keyboard.

You know your keyboard is too low when you have to bend your forearms or wrists downward to use it, or when you have to bend your head and neck forward and downward to see it. If your keyboard is too low and is not adjustable, raise it to just below your hand level by placing it on books, so that your fingers automatically rest on the third row of keys from the bottom of the keyboard.

Your keyboard is too high if you have to hunch up your shoulders and bend your wrists upward with your fingers bending downward, or if you have to bend your forearms upward with your wrists bent downward in order to rest your fingers on it. Repeatedly lifting your shoulders or bending your forearms and wrists will strain your upper back and neck muscles.

If you presently place your keyboard on the writing surface of your desk, causing the keyboard to sit too high, consider buying a keyboard tray [511], which can be installed below your writing surface at slightly below elbow level. A keyboard tray will place your keyboard at the correct height to match the ideal computer posture previously described in this chapter. It will also bring the keyboard and mouse closer to your body, which keeps your forearms from resting on the hard edge of your desk.

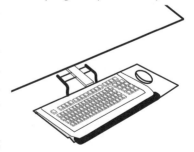

Keyboard on Keyboard Tray

A common mistake is placing the keyboard too far away from your body, forcing you to extend your arms to reach it. This constant stretching can strain your upper back and neck muscles. The keyboard should be placed in a position that allows you to maintain the proper posture previously described.

THE TILT OF YOUR KEYBOARD

If you have a normal-size hand, never place your keyboard flat! The back of your keyboard should be raised so that the keyboard is angled slightly toward you. This allows you to get closer to your work without bending your head and neck forward and downward. Use the built-in risers under the back of the keyboard to raise it. If your keyboard does not come with such a propping mechanism, place a few magazines or a thin book under the back of it to tilt it.

However, if you have large hands or long fingers, place your keyboard flat. This will prevent you from having to bend your wrists upward and your fingers downward to reach the keys, compressing the structures in your wrists.

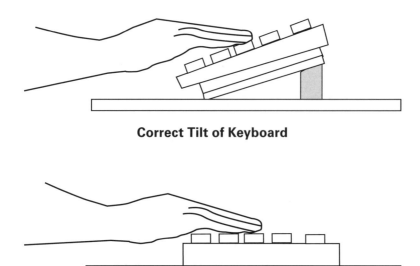

Correct Tilt of Keyboard

Position of Keyboard When You Have Long Fingers

UNSTABLE OR WOBBLY KEYBOARDS

An unstable or wobbly keyboard will cause you to assume a locked, strained posture and will force you to pound on the keys with a lot of force to keep the keyboard in place. Putting heavy pressure on the keys stresses your upper back and neck muscles.

WIRELESS KEYBOARDS

Wireless keyboards [521] are excellent for maintaining correct posture. You can place a wireless keyboard in your lap—a more natural position than placing it on a desk.

ERGONOMIC KEYBOARDS

The typical computer keyboard is rectangular and does not align properly with the human body. Your shoulders are wider than a computer keyboard, and when you place your fingers on a standard keyboard, you have to angle your forearms inward and bend your wrists sideways to align your fingers to the keys, straining your wrists.

When wrists are repeatedly bent in an unnatural posture, pressure builds up on the blood vessels and nerves that go into the hands, causing carpal tunnel syndrome. An ergonomic keyboard [522] is excellent at preventing this condition because its typing surface is angled to align with the natural posture of your hands and arms, thus relieving the strains to your wrists.

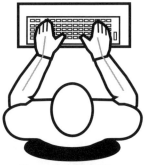

**Harmful Position
of Wrists**

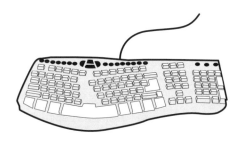

Ergonomic Keyboard

MOUSE PLACEMENT

The correct location of your mouse is right next to your keyboard on the side of your primary hand. The mouse should always be within easy reach of your primary hand. If you place the mouse further back than your keyboard, you will be forced to stretch to reach for it, pulling on your neck and shoulder muscles.

WRIST SUPPORTS

In order for your wrists to be in a neutral position—not bent up or down or twisted to the side—they must be in line with your forearms. To help your wrists maintain this neutral position, use a wrist support.

A wrist support is an oblong object approximately one inch thick, eighteen inches long, and four inches wide. Place the wrist support at the same height as your keyboard. When your wrists are supported, your neck and shoulder muscles can relax more too.

For best results, use a padded wrist support[523] or gel-filled wrist support[524] that is not too hard or too soft. Using a wrist support that is too hard is like resting your wrist on a sharp object, which compresses the contents of your wrists. This is the opposite effect a wrist support was designed to have. A too-soft wrist support allows your wrists to sag, also compressing the contents of your wrists and making it more difficult to move your hands. When your hands are not freely moveable as you type, you will bend your wrists to the side, straining them.

Gently rest your wrists on the wrist support, rather than leaning on it. Leaning on a wrist support will strain your wrists, arms, shoulder and neck muscles, and, as noted, will also compress the contents of your wrists, leading to carpal tunnel syndrome.

The neck-aids and neck-appliances described in this chapter can be ordered through your family chiropractor or from the Neck and Back Products store at **www.NeckAndBackProducts.com** or call toll-free **1-800-882-4476**.

15

Neck-Proofing Your Workplace When You Have a Standing Occupation

Many of the rules that apply to neck-proofing sitting occupations also apply to standing occupations. As a brief refresher, correct standing posture is when:

- You are standing straight without bending your neck.

- You are facing forward with your eyes and feet pointed straight ahead.

- The object you are looking at is clearly visible by looking straight ahead or by simply tilting your eyes "up" or "down."

- Your ear hole, mid shoulder, mid hip, and ankles are in a straight vertical line when viewed from the side.

- Your shoulders are resting comfortably on top of your rib cage.

- Your upper arms are hanging straight down.

- Your lower arms can be bent at right angles to your upper arm, parallel to the floor to reach the objects you intend to use.

- Your hands and wrists are in line with your lower arms.

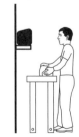

Correct Standing Work Posture

- Your lower back is slightly arched forward.
- Your neck, shoulders, arms, and lower back are relaxed.

Standing Work Neck Rules

STANDING WORK NECK RULE #1:
Keep your neck as still as possible; do not quickly bend your neck upward or downward, or turn it.
A sudden bending or turning of your neck can injure your neck muscles and spinal joints.

STANDING WORK NECK RULE #2:
Always face your work.
Facing your work prevents you from having to keep your neck in a turned position for prolonged periods.

STANDING WORK NECK RULE #3:
While maintaining correct posture and without bending your neck, look straight ahead or simply raise or lower your eyes to view objects as needed. The goal is to keep your head directly over your shoulders.

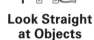

Look Straight at Objects

STANDING WORK NECK RULE #4:
Use work surfaces that match your occupation.
To keep you from constantly bending your head and neck downward to look at your work, any objects you are working on should be between your waist and shoulder level.

Because people are different shapes and sizes and have different occupations, their work surfaces must match their bodies and their types of tasks. You will need to adjust your work surfaces to fit your body and the type of work you do; otherwise, your body will automatically adjust to fit your work environment—usually creating strains in your neck.

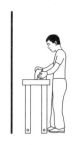

Place Work Objects between Waist and Shoulders

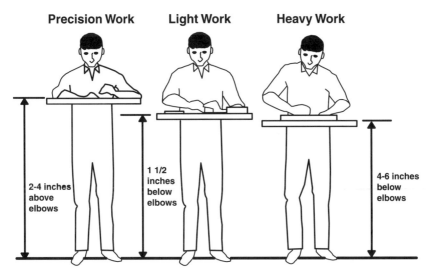

Precision Work   Light Work   Heavy Work

2-4 inches above elbows

1 1/2 inches below elbows

4-6 inches below elbows

Height of Work Surfaces

If your job entails precision work, your work surface should be two to four inches above your elbows.

If you do light work, your standing work counter should be one and a half inches below your elbows.

If your standing occupation requires lifting heavy objects from your work surface, your work surface should be four to six inches below your elbows.

STANDING WORK NECK RULE #5:
Do not maintain a bent-forward posture.
Maintaining a bent-forward posture reverses the normal curve of your neck, straining it.

STANDING WORK NECK RULE #6:
Avoid prolonged bending, leaning, or rotating of your neck.
Avoid leaning your head to the side (e.g., cradling a telephone between your head and shoulder) or being bent forward over a work surface for long periods of time. When neck muscles are in one posture too long, the blood flow to these muscles is restricted. With less blood, muscles tighten and produce pain. When one neck muscle begins to hurt, its neighboring muscles tighten to help support the weight of the head. Then these

225

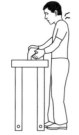 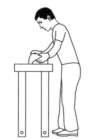 

Avoid Prolonged Bending of Neck   **Don't Maintain a Bent-Forward Posture**   **Prolonged Leaning of Neck**

muscles begin to hurt, which causes other muscles to tighten, and so on. The final result is a lot of pain!

STANDING WORK NECK RULE #7:
Alternate the direction in which your neck and back are bending.
Some occupations require you to hold your neck or back in a single position for a prolonged period of time (e.g., bending, leaning, etc.). If this is the case with your work, make every effort to alternate your position every ten minutes—lean first to the right for ten minutes, then lean to the left for ten minutes, and so on.

STANDING WORK NECK RULE #8:
Minimize stretching to reach for work objects.
Whenever you overstretch to reach for objects, your arm and upper shoulder muscles pull on your neck, causing a strain to your upper back and neck muscles.

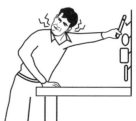

Don't Overstretch

STANDING WORK NECK RULE #9:
Take frequent stretch breaks.
Be sure to take a brief rest period from your work every hour. Standing in one position for long periods of time places a tremendous amount of stress on your neck and shoulder muscles, restricting the blood flow to these muscles. To counter this muscle damage, move around once every hour and go through three or four range-of-motion exercises (see Chapter 16). These exercises will increase the circulation to your muscles, relaxing

them. The exercises will also return the circulation to the discs of your neck, helping prevent a disc injury.

Standing Work Ergonomics

ERGONOMICALLY ADJUSTABLE STANDING WORK SURFACES

Some places of employment have work surfaces that can be adjusted upward or downward, or that can be tilted to match the different heights of their employees. If your standing work surface is adjustable, follow the guidelines of this chapter to raise, lower, or tilt it to the level that is right for you. However, most work surfaces are not adjustable; thus, they have to be modified to become the ideal height for each individual.

THE HEIGHT OF YOUR WORK SURFACE

If your body is not comfortable using a work surface at its present height, you will need to raise or lower the surface until you are able to maintain normal posture with your neck and shoulders relaxed.

Most standing work surfaces are too low. You know that your work surface is too low if you have to bend forward excessively to view your work. If your work surface is too low and is not adjustable, you can place a large, thick wooden chopping block on top of your work surface to raise it to the desired level. Also place a desk shelf[506] on the back of your work surface to raise your materials higher.

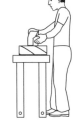

Raising Work Surface

You know your work surface is too high if you have to hunch your shoulders upward to work. If this is the case, lower your work surface to the proper level. If your work surface is not adjustable, raise your body in relationship to the work surface by building a riser, or a long, thin box, that is of sufficient height to allow you to maintain normal posture while working. The riser should be as long as your workstation, four to five feet wide, and covered with a non-slip surface. Sitting on a perch chair (like a bar stool) that promotes a sort of sit-stand posture is an acceptable alternative.

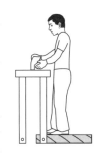

Stand on Riser

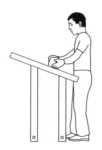
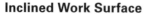
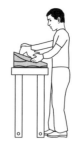

Inclined Work Surface   **Inclined Riser**

THE INCLINE OF YOUR WORK SURFACE

Always do your best to avoid working with your head and neck bent forward. One way to do this is to incline your workbench or table ten to fifteen degrees downward toward you. Tilting your work surface toward you helps take the strain off of your neck.

If your work surface is unable to be tilted, build a new work surface the same measurements as your existing work surface but with the front of it ten to fifteen degrees lower than the back. Place the new work surface on top of the old work surface.

THE PLACEMENT OF OBJECTS ON YOUR STANDING WORK SURFACE

Always strive to keep your body in a straight, strain-free posture. Usually you can accomplish this by keeping your work surface and reading heights at their proper levels and the items you most frequently use within easy reach from your body.

The objects you use the most should be placed directly in front of you, within twenty inches of your body. The objects you use somewhat less

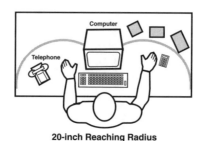

20-inch Reaching Radius

Ergonomic Placement of Work Objects

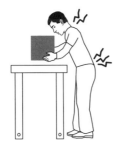

**Don't Stretch When
Lifting Heavy Objects**

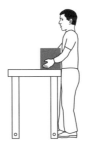

**Position Yourself Close to
Heavy Objects Before Lifting**

frequently should be placed within the same twenty-inch distance, but on the side of your primary hand and slightly to the side of the objects you use most. Place even less frequently used objects within the same twenty-inch reaching distance, but on the side of your non-primary hand.

If you must lift heavy objects from your work surface, always place them at the front of the work surface before lifting them in order to prevent stretching forward to lift them. The farther away an object to be lifted is, the easier it is to strain your neck.

IF YOUR STANDING OCCUPATION REQUIRES FREQUENT FORWARD REACHING

To avoid excessive forward reaching, place all objects you frequently use in front of you within twenty inches of your body.

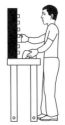

**Place Objects
Within Easy Reach**

IF YOUR STANDING OCCUPATION REQUIRES FREQUENT READING

You never want to bend over to read while working. In order to avoid this, place your reading material above your workbench at slightly below eye level. If the written material you frequently view is placed too low, it will force you to bend your head and neck forward and downward to read it, straining your neck muscles. One solution is to place the material in a raised document holder [525] or slantboard [503], again, at slightly below eye level.

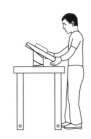

**Document
Holder on Stand**

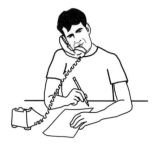

**Cradling Telephone
Causes Neck Strain**

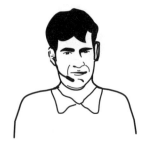

Hands-Free Headset

IF YOUR STANDING OCCUPATION REQUIRES FREQUENT USE OF THE TELEPHONE

If your job requires you to use a telephone more than 20 percent of the day, get a hands-free headset [508], a speakerphone [501], or a built-up phone handle [509] to reduce the strain on your neck and to eliminate the headaches caused by cradling the phone between your head and shoulder. Headsets and speakerphones also free your hands to simultaneously conduct other work while using the telephone with your head and neck in a normal posture.

IF YOUR STANDING OCCUPATION REQUIRES THE USE OF A COMPUTER

If you use a computer in your standing occupation and the computer screen you frequently view is placed too low, it will force you to bend your head and neck forward and downward to read the screen, straining your neck. If so, raise your screen to the correct eye level by placing it on a "riser" [515] or large computer base.

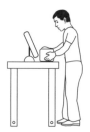

**Computer Screen Placement
Too Low**

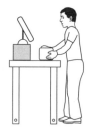

Place Computer on Riser

If you use a computer at your standing workstation, follow the instructions in Chapter 14 about how to set up a computer workstation with the proper positioning of items on your work surface.

IF YOUR STANDING OCCUPATION REQUIRES YOU TO CONSTANTLY LOOK UPWARD

If you find yourself constantly looking upward in your work (e.g., to see a computer screen), you are likely to develop an overuse syndrome of your neck, which causes pain.

If you have to repeatedly tilt your head upward to view objects, the objects are placed too high. To solve the problem, lower any objects you frequently view. This benefits you by reducing the number of times you have to look upward for prolonged periods of time.

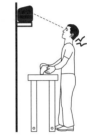

Computer Screen Placement - Too High

If for some reason you cannot lower these objects, raise your standing height by building a box that is the length of your work surface area, approximately four to six feet wide, and of sufficient height to raise you to the desired eye level. The surface of the box should be covered with a non-slip material to prevent you from slipping.

Once you have raised your body to the proper eye level, raise your work surface to the proper level, if necessary, by following the instructions given earlier in this chapter in the section "The Height of Your Work Surface."

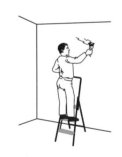

Stand on Stepladder

If you only occasionally have to look upward to do overhead work, stand on a ladder or step stool [406] to face your work.

IF YOU WEAR BIFOCAL OR TRIFOCAL GLASSES

Sometimes wearing bifocals or trifocals causes a person to tilt his or her head upward to view an object. In this case, the object to be viewed may not be too high. Rather, the tilting of the head is due to the glasses, not the object's height. If you find yourself tilting your head upward to see through your glasses, you can buy special single-vision computer glasses where the entire glass magnifies objects the same amount, thus reducing the necessity of tilting your head upward.

Wearing bifocal or trifocal glasses when walking is dangerous because you will have to bend your head and neck downward to see the ground clearly, which can strain your neck muscles. If your occupation requires substantial walking, consider purchasing "walking glasses" or glasses with a different prescription for each eye.

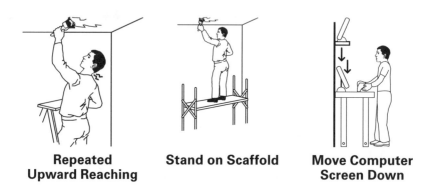

Repeated Upward Reaching   **Stand on Scaffold**   **Move Computer Screen Down**

IF YOUR STANDING OCCUPATION REQUIRES CONSTANT UPWARD REACHING

Repeatedly reaching upward places your neck in excessive backward bending, straining your neck muscles and compressing the joints at the back of your neck. Instead of reaching upward, move the objects you frequently have to reach for down to your waist level. If your occupation requires frequent overhead reaching, such as with a painter or plasterer, use a ladder or scaffolding and move it often to stay close to your work.

STANDING ON HARD SURFACES

Standing on hard surfaces produces a strain on your back and neck. When possible, stand on an anti-fatigue rubber mat[526] or carpet to relieve the strain.

STORAGE OF MATERIALS IN STANDING OCCUPATIONS

Store frequently used items between elbow and shoulder height to minimize bending your neck or reaching overhead. Store rarely used and lighter objects above your work surface and store heavy objects at floor

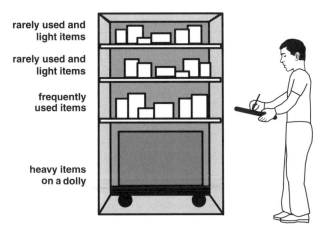

"Body to Storage Area" Relationship

level. If an object is very heavy, place it on a dolly that has wheels so that you can move it easily.

PROLONGED STANDING

When standing for long periods of time, transfer your weight from one foot to the other or alternate placing each foot on a step stool [406] or foot rail. Putting one foot on a step stool or foot rail places your lower back in a normal forward curve, relaxing it. This automatically creates a desired forward curve in your neck and thus relieves stress on your neck too.

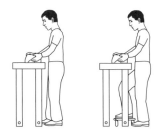

Place Foot on Step Stool

Better yet, instead of standing all day, alternate between standing and sitting on a tall chair such as a bar stool. This alternation will reduce your back and neck strain.

Section Four:

Creating a Strong Neck

16

Exercising Your Way to a Healthy, Strong Neck

The key to a healthy, functioning neck is vertebrae that are correctly aligned and freely movable, surrounded by strong supporting neck muscles. To correct the alignment and mobility of your vertebrae, you will need the care of a chiropractor. To strengthen your neck muscles, you will need to follow a sensible exercise program. By getting chiropractic adjustments (spinal manipulations) and doing stretching and strengthening exercises, you can almost always maintain a pain-free neck.

Exercising your neck increases the circulation of blood to your muscles, restores muscle strength, increases neck flexibility, and helps maintain the normal range of motion of your neck vertebrae.

Neck Exercises

SAFETY GUIDELINES FOR EXERCISING YOUR NECK

1. **Only do exercises that are appropriate for <u>you</u>.**

   Before beginning this exercise program, show this book to your chiropractor and have him or her specify which exercises you need to do. Also have your chiropractor recommend the frequency (how often) and number of repetitions (how many) for each exercise.

Ask your chiropractor to place a "✔" in the appropriate box "❏" located at the beginning of each exercise.

2. **Do not start a neck exercise program if you are in pain, unless instructed to do so by your chiropractor.**

3. **Do not exercise immediately after a chiropractic adjustment (<u>spinal</u> manipulation).** Wait at least four to six hours.

4. **Do your exercises daily.** Exercising with regularity strengthens your neck muscles more quickly.

5. **Work your way into exercising. In other words, do not attempt to start all of these exercises at the same time.** Studies have shown that when people attempt to do too many exercises too soon, they will usually quit. Start with the easy stretching exercises. Then, when you have gotten familiar with those, add the strengthening exercises. The stretching exercises prepare your muscles for the strengthening exercises.

6. **Do not try to accomplish too much in a single exercise session.** When exercising, start your routine slowly and then gradually increase the intensity. The permanent strengthening of your neck muscles is a slow process that cannot be hurried.

7. **All exercise movements should be smooth, not jerky.** Any sudden movement while exercising can injure your muscles.

8. **Exercise only to the "point of pain." Do not *cause* pain or discomfort.** The phrase "no pain, no gain" does not apply to spinal exercises. When you start your exercises, feeling a small amount of discomfort is normal. However, your exercises should not produce pain that lingers after you have stopped exercising nor should they cause a symptom (e.g., arm pain or numbness in your hands). As soon as you experience any pain or other symptoms, stop the exercise. Again, the idea is to exercise to the point of pain or discomfort, not to *cause* pain or discomfort.

People who exercise just to the point of pain and who avoid over-exercising by listening to their body's **neck-talk**, strengthen their neck muscles more quickly than the "hero" who tries to "work through the pain." "Working through the pain" creates serious risk of injury.

9. **Exercise your neck, shoulder, and mid back areas together.** Whenever you stretch and strengthen your neck muscles, you always need to stretch and strengthen your shoulder and mid back muscles as well, because all of these areas are interconnected. Attempting to correct or strengthen one area without correcting or strengthening the other areas does not work. All three areas must be corrected or strengthened at the same time.

10. **Always *stretch* your neck, shoulders, and mid back first, then *strengthen*.** Once you have completed the stretching exercises for all three areas, follow with the strengthening exercises for all three. Do not stretch and strengthen the neck, then stretch and strengthen the mid back, and so on. The strengthening exercises of one area will interfere with the stretching of the other areas.

11. **If any exercise hurts your neck, stop immediately—pain is an indication that you are injuring yourself.**

"Which Exercises Should I Do?"

Do two or three of each neck, shoulder, and mid back stretching exercise prescribed in this chapter, followed by two or three repetitions of each strengthening exercise for these areas. Then, gradually increase the number of repetitions of each stretching and strengthening exercise.

Neck Stretching Exercises

It is important to stretch your muscles before strengthening them. When neck muscles are too tight, normal neck movements pull on them throughout the day. The neck muscles respond to this pulling by tightening even more, straining the muscles and possibly pulling the neck vertebrae out of alignment. Stretching loosens the tension within the muscles and lubricates the joints of the neck. However, there is a big difference between loosening the tight tissues of your neck and overstretching them. Stretching helps the muscles; overstretching hurts them.

Motion of the neck is measured in two ways—active and passive. Each joint in your body has its active range of motion. For instance, turn your head as far to one side as it will go. This distance is your neck's active range of rotation movement, or range of motion. Almost all exercises occur within your active range of motion. However, if you use your hand to press gently on your head, you will be able to turn your neck a little further. This further rotation is considered your neck's passive range of motion. Passive ranges of motion are almost always greater than active ranges of motion.

The following exercises will increase both the active and passive ranges of motion in your neck. These exercises stretch tight muscles and ligaments, re-establishing your neck's normal range of motion.

But before we start stretching, let us establish some rules for doing so safely and for getting the most benefit from your stretching exercises.

NECK STRETCHING RULES

1. With every neck stretching exercise, try to increase the range of motion of your neck in each direction.

2. Stretch only until you feel a mild tension, and not pain, in your muscles.

3. The feeling of the stretch should slightly subside as you hold the stretch.

4. If the feeling of the stretch increases in intensity as you hold the stretch, gently back off. An increase in intensity indicates that you are overstretching.

5. Never bounce your muscles while performing stretching exercises; bouncing may injure your muscles.

6. If a stretching exercise produces pain, cease it immediately. Pain indicates that muscles are being strained.

7. If you are suffering from neck pain, only do these stretching exercises under the prescription of your chiropractor.

As noted, the following neck stretching exercises should be performed two to three times a day, with two to three repetitions each time, before performing any neck strengthening exercises. Gradually increase these stretching exercises to ten times a day with ten repetitions each time. Children under twelve should do only one to two repetitions of these stretches three times a day.

REMINDER: Do stretching exercises for all three areas—neck, shoulders, and mid back—before moving on to any strengthening exercises.

NECK STRETCHING EXERCISE #1:

Forward Bending Neck Stretch: This exercise will increase the forward bending of your neck and is especially helpful in relieving headaches.

Doctor's prescription:

❑   Do this stretching exercise _____ times a day with _____ repetitions each time.

Instructions:

- In a sitting position, look straight ahead.

- Start with your chin and head level.

- Tuck in your chin. This will prevent compression of your nerve roots.

- Keep your shoulders level.

- Interlace your fingers behind your mid neck, not your head. Or, grasp each end of a "Posture Pulley" [300] and place it behind your mid neck.

- Drop your head forward and downward with your chin toward your chest as far as possible. Let gravity help pull your head down, stretching your neck even further.

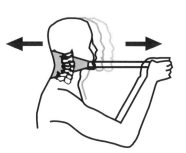

Utilize a Posture Pulley

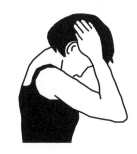

"Forward-Bending" Neck Stretching Exercise Incorrect Hand Placement

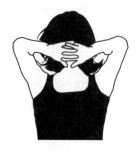

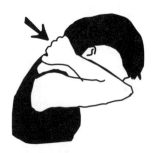

"Forward-Bending" **Correct Hand Placement**
Neck Stretching Exercise

- Relax your arms while pointing your elbows downward, allowing the weight of your arms to pull your head even further downward.

- Then, using your interlaced fingers or "Posture Pulley," gently but firmly pull your head and neck into further forward bending, up to your tolerance.

- Hold your head and neck in this forward position for eight to ten seconds.

- Then, *slowly* return your head and neck to the normal position. If you return to the starting position too quickly, your muscles will act like a stretched rubber band that is suddenly released and will contract too quickly, producing pain.

> **CAUTION:** Make sure you do not grab your *head* and pull it forward, as this can cause or increase a head-forward posture. If your neck vertebrae are in an abnormally straightened or reversed position, only do this exercise under a chiropractor's prescription.

NECK STRETCHING EXERCISE #2:
Backward Bending Neck Stretch: This exercise stretches the muscles and ligaments of the front of your neck.

Doctor's prescription:
❏   Do this stretching exercise _____ times a day with _____ repetitions each time.

Instructions:

- In a sitting position, look straight ahead.

- Start with your chin and head level.

- Keep your shoulders level.

- Place your fingers under your chin.

- Bend your head and neck slowly backward as far as possible as if looking up
at the ceiling. Let gravity help pull
your head down to stretch your neck
even further.

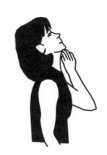

**"Backward-Bending"
Neck Stretching
Exercise**

- Then, using your fingers, gently push your head and neck further
backward as far as possible, up to your tolerance.

- Hold your head and neck in this backward position for eight to
ten seconds.

- Then slowly return your head and neck to the starting position.

NECK STRETCHING EXERCISE #3:

Sideways Bending Neck Stretch: This exercise stretches the muscles
and ligaments of the sides of your neck. The muscles of the sides of the
neck are especially prone to becoming tight in people who frequently
tense their upper shoulder muscles (e.g., typists, computer operators, etc.).
People with headaches, and jaw pain usually find this exercise beneficial
in relieving their pain.

Doctor's prescription:

❏ Do this stretching exercise _____ times a day with _____ repetitions
each time.

Instructions:

- In a sitting position, look straight ahead.

- Start with your chin and head level.

- Tuck your chin in. This will prevent compression of your nerve roots.

- Keep your shoulders down and relaxed.

- Place your right hand over the top of your head with your fingers touching above your left ear.

- Tilt your head to the right as far as it will go while keeping your gaze forward, let the weight of your head pull it further downward.

- Then, using two of the fingers of your right hand, pull your head and neck to the right as far as possible, within reason, so that your right ear approaches your right shoulder.

- Make sure you do not bring your left shoulder up to your ear. Do so by holding on to the left side of the chair with your left hand. And, do not allow your head to turn as you perform this exercise (i.e., do not bring your nose to your shoulder). The turning of your head when performing this exercise will compress the nerves of your neck. You are attempting to touch your ear, not your nose, to your shoulder.

"Sideways-Bending" Neck Stretching Exercise

- Hold your head and neck in this sideways position for eight to ten seconds.

- Then, slowly return to the starting position.

- Repeat this exercise on the left side using the left hand to pull your head to the left. At the same time, hold on to the right side of the chair with your right hand.

   CAUTION: As this exercise is simple to do, it is also easy to overdo. Therefore, proceed slowly and carefully.

NECK STRETCHING EXERCISE #4:
Rotation (Head Turning) Neck Stretch: This exercise stretches the muscles and ligaments that affect the turning of the neck.

Doctor's prescription:
❑   Do this stretching exercise _____ times a day with _____ repetitions each time.

Instructions:

- In a sitting position, look straight ahead.

- Keep your chin and head level.

- Tuck your chin in. This will prevent compression of your nerve roots.

- Turn your head as far to the right as possible, as if you are going to look over your right shoulder.

- Place the fingers of your left hand along the left side of your cheekbone and gently help push your head further to the right.

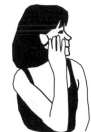

- Hold your head and neck in this rotated position for eight to ten seconds.

- Then, slowly return to the starting position.

- Repeat this stretching exercise on the left side, using the fingers of the right hand.

"Rotation of Neck" Stretching Exercise

NECK STRETCHING EXERCISE #5:

Head and Neck Rolling Stretch: This exercise stretches the muscles and ligaments that affect the leaning and turning of the neck.

Doctor's prescription:
❑ Do this stretching exercise _____ times a day with _____ repetitions each time.

Instructions:

- In a sitting position, look straight ahead.

- Start with your chin and head level.

- Keep your shoulders level. Try not to let your shoulders drift up to your ears.

- Tilt your head to the right side as far as it will go.

- Roll your head forward and down, attempting to touch your chin to your chest.

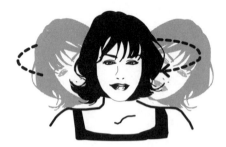

"Head Rolling" Neck Stretching Exercise

- Continue this rolling motion to the left as if attempting to touch your left ear to your left shoulder.

- Then, continue rolling your head in a full circle by tilting your head backward.

- Then, slowly return to the starting position.

- Repeat this exercise to your left.

> **CAUTION:** If you have neck pain, only do this exercise under the prescription of your chiropractor. Rolling your head in a circle can aggravate a neck problem. As with any exercise, if you feel pain doing this exercise, discontinue it.

Neck Strengthening Exercises

Perform the previous range-of-motion stretching exercises until you have achieved normal range of motion in your neck. Then add resistance to each exercise with your hands, progressively adding stronger resistance until you can totally stop the motion of your head and neck without feeling discomfort. These "range of motion against resistance" exercises build strength.

The following neck strengthening exercises should be performed two to three times a day, with two to three repetitions each time, only after you have performed the neck stretching exercises. Gradually increase these strengthening exercises to ten times a day with ten repetitions each time. Children under twelve should do only one to two repetitions of these exercises three times a day.

CAUTION: If you have neck pain or a neck strain, only do these resistance exercises under the prescription of your chiropractor.

NECK STRENGTHENING EXERCISE #1:

Forward Bending Neck Strengthener: This exercise strengthens the muscles of the front of your neck.

Doctor's prescription:

☐ Do this strengthening exercise ＿＿ times a day with ＿＿ repetitions each time.

Instructions:

- In a sitting position, look straight ahead.
- Start with your chin and head level.
- Tuck in your chin. This will prevent compression of your nerve roots.
- Keep your shoulders level.
- Place the palms of your hands over both sides of your face.
- Press your head against your palms, then bend your head and neck forward and downward against the gentle resistance of your hands.

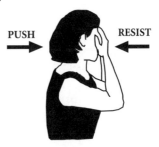

"Forward-Bending" Neck Strengthening Exercise

- Hold your head and neck in the forward position, against resistance, for eight to ten seconds.
- Then, slowly return to the starting position.
- Gradually increase the resistance of each exercise.

NECK STRENGTHENING EXERCISE #2:

Backward Bending Neck Strengthener: This exercise strengthens the muscles of the back of your neck.

Doctor's prescription:

❑ Do this strengthening exercise _____ times a day with _____ repetitions each time.

Instructions:

- In a sitting position, look straight ahead.

- Start with your chin and head level.

- Tuck your chin in. This will prevent compression of your nerve roots.

- Keep your shoulders level.

- Interlock your fingers at the back of your mid neck, not behind your head. A "Posture Pulley" [300] can be used instead of interlocking your fingers.

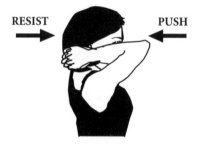

- Bend your head and neck backward and slightly downward against the gentle resistance of your hands or the "Posture Pulley."

"Backward-Bending"
Neck Strengthening Exercise

- Hold your head and neck in the backward position, against resistance, for eight to ten seconds.

- Then, slowly return to the starting position.

- Gradually increase the resistance of each exercise.

    CAUTION: Your interlocked fingers or the "Posture Pulley" should be behind your neck, not against the back of your head. Placing resistance in an incorrect position can make a head-forward posture worse.

NECK STRENGTHENING EXERCISE #3:

Sideways Bending Neck Strengthener: This exercise strengthens the muscles of the side of your neck.

Doctor's prescription:

❑ Do this strengthening exercise _____ times a day with _____ repetitions each time.

Instructions:

- In a sitting position, look straight ahead.

- Start with your chin and head level.

- Tuck your chin in. This will prevent compression of your nerve roots.

- Keep your shoulders level.

- Place your right hand against the right side of your head above the ear, with your fingers pointing upward.

- Lean your head toward your right shoulder, against the resistance of your right hand.

- Hold your head and neck in this sideways position, against resistance, for eight to ten seconds.

- Then, slowly return to the starting position.

- Repeat this exercise on your left side using your left hand.

- Gradually increase the resistance of each exercise.

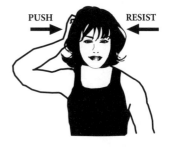

"Sideways-Bending" Neck Strengthening Exercise

CAUTION: Do not allow your head to turn as you perform this exercise (i.e., do not bring your nose to your shoulder). Turning your head when performing this exercise can compress the nerves of your neck.

NECK STRENGTHENING EXERCISE #4:

Rotation (Head Turning) Neck Strengthener: This exercise strengthens the muscles that turn your neck.

Doctor's prescription:

☐ Do this strengthening exercise _____ times a day with _____ repetitions each time.

Instructions:

- In a sitting position, look straight ahead.

- Start with your chin and head level.

- Tuck your chin in. This will prevent compression of your nerve roots.

- Keep your shoulders level.

- Place your right hand against your right temple.

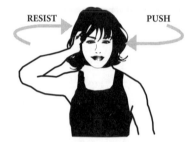

"Rotation of Neck" Strengthening Exercise

- Rotate your head to the right, against the gentle resistance of your right hand.

- Hold your head and neck in the rotated position, against resistance, for eight to ten seconds.

- Then, slowly return to the starting position.

- Repeat this exercise on your left side using your left hand.

- Gradually increase the resistance of each exercise.

Neck Strengthening Exercises Using a Neck Strengthening Device

It is important to follow the manufacturer's directions for placing the neck strengthening device on your head and securing the resistance bands to a door frame or wall. The following is an example of how these neck strengthening aids are used.

NECK STRENGTHENING EXERCISE #5:

Front of Neck Strengthener Using a Neck Strengthening Device [301]:
This exercise strengthens the muscles at the front of your neck.

Doctor's prescription:
☐   Do this strengthening exercise _____ times a day with _____ repetitions each time.

Instructions:
- Stand facing away from a wall or door, within eight inches of the wall or door.
- Look straight ahead.
- Place your chin, head, and shoulders in a level position.
- Push your head forward and slightly downward against the resistance of the neck strengthening device.
- Start with minimum pull strength, then gradually increase the pull strength with each exercise.
- Hold your pressure against the pull of the neck strengthening device for eight to ten seconds.
- Then, slowly return to the beginning position.

   NOTE: This exercise aid can be used to enhance the other neck exercises described in this chapter.

NECK STRENGTHENING EXERCISE #6:

Back of Neck Strengthener Using a Neck Strengthening Device:
This exercise strengthens the muscles at the back of your neck.

Doctor's prescription:
☐   Do this strengthening exercise _____ times a day with _____ repetitions each time.

Instructions:
- Stand facing a wall or door, within eight inches of the wall or door.
- Look straight ahead.
- Place your chin, head, and shoulders in a level position.

- Push your head backward against the resistance of the neck strengthening device.

- Start with minimum pull strength, then gradually increase the pull strength with each exercise.

- Hold your pressure against the pull of the neck strengthening device for eight to ten seconds.

- Then, slowly return to the starting position.

NECK STRENGTHENING EXERCISE #7:
Side of the Neck Strengthener Using a Neck Strengthening Device:
This exercise strengthens the muscles of the side of your neck.

Doctor's prescription:
❑ Do this strengthening exercise _____ times a day with _____ repetitions each time.

Instructions:
- Stand with your right shoulder touching a wall or door. Your body is at right angles to the wall or door.

- Look straight ahead.

- Place your chin, head, and shoulders in a level position.

- Push your head to the left and slightly downward, against the resistance of the neck strengthening device.

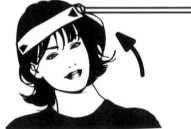

Neck Strengthening Device

- Start with minimum pull strength, then gradually increase the pull strength with each exercise.

- Hold your pressure against the pull of the neck strengthening device for eight to ten seconds.

- Then, slowly return to the starting position.

- Repeat this exercise with your left shoulder against a wall or door, bending your head to the right.

SHOULDER EXERCISES

To completely strengthen the neck, it is necessary to loosen and then strengthen the shoulder area as well. The reason for this is that whenever the muscles and ligaments of the shoulders are tight, they will pull on your neck, preventing your neck from becoming totally stretched and strengthened. Loosening the shoulder muscles and ligaments relaxes their pull on your neck area, allowing your neck to become stronger and to return to its normal, healthy posture.

Once your shoulders are loosened, you can then maintain them in their normal position by doing shoulder strengthening exercises.

Shoulder Stretching Exercises

The following shoulder stretching exercises should be performed two to three times a day, with two to three repetitions each time. Gradually increase these exercises to ten times a day with ten repetitions each time. Children under twelve should do only one to two repetitions of these exercises three times a day.

SHOULDER STRETCHING EXERCISE #1:

The "Trap" Muscles Stretch: This maneuver stretches the muscles and ligaments of the sides of the neck and the trapezius muscle. The trapezius muscle is the large diamond-shaped muscle that starts at the back of your head, extends outward to your shoulder joints, and then to the middle of your mid back.

Doctor's prescription:

❏ Do this stretching exercise _____ times a day with _____ repetitions each time.

Instructions:

- Stand or sit up straight in a chair that supports your mid back.
- Look straight ahead.
- Start with your head, ears, and chin level.
- Keep your arms hanging at your sides.

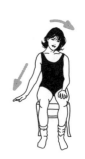

- To stretch the right side of your neck, lean your left ear toward your left shoulder as far as possible.

- Then, force your right shoulder downward while reaching down your side with your right arm.

- At the same time, turn your face slightly to the left.

- Hold this position for eight to ten seconds.

- Then, slowly return to the starting position.

- Repeat this stretching exercise on the opposite side.

"Trap Stretching" Exercise

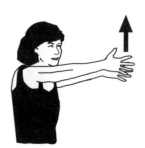 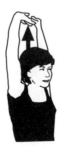 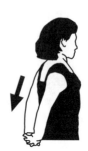

"Front of Shoulder" Stretching Exercise

SHOULDER STRETCHING EXERCISE #2:
Front of Shoulders Stretch: This exercise stretches, relaxes, and loosens the front of your shoulders, and is specifically necessary if you have the habit of slumping your shoulders forward.

Doctor's prescription:
❑ Do this stretching exercise _____ times a day with _____ repetitions each time.

Instructions:
- Stand up straight.
- Keep your head level.

- Starting with your arms at your sides, swing your arms forward, then upward toward the ceiling.

- Then, interlock your fingers and turn your palms upward toward the ceiling with your thumbs facing forward. At the same time, try to lengthen your arms toward the ceiling.

- Hold this position for eight to ten seconds.

- Then, keeping your elbows behind the midline of the side of your body, lower your arms as though you are putting your hands into your back pockets.

- When your hands reach your back pockets, bring your hands together, interlocking the fingers of both hands.

- Then, slowly straighten both arms while turning both elbows inward as far as they will go. At the same time, stretch your arms downward as far as they will go.

- Hold this position for eight to ten seconds.

- Then, while your hands remain clasped, bring both hands and arms backward and upward toward the ceiling as far as they can go.

- Then, slowly return to the starting position.

SHOULDER STRETCHING EXERCISE #3:
The "Behind Your Head" Stretch: This exercise stretches the muscles and ligaments that control the upward motion of your shoulders.

Doctor's prescription:
❑ Do this stretching exercise _____ times a day with _____ repetitions each time.

Instructions:
- Stand or sit up straight in a chair that supports your mid back.

- Keep your head straight upward with your head and chin level.

- Reach straight upward with your right arm.

- Bending at the elbow, bring your right forearm downward attempting to reach the mid portion of your upper back.

- Grab your right elbow with your left hand.

- Gently pull your right elbow behind your head as far as it will go.

- Hold this position for eight to ten seconds.

- Then, slowly return to your starting position.

- Repeat this exercise on your left shoulder.

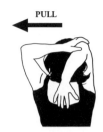

PULL

"Behind Your Head" Stretching Exercise

Shoulder Stretching and Strengthening Exercises

These exercises loosen overly tight shoulder muscles and ligaments, allowing the shoulders to return to their normal function. These exercises also strengthen the shoulder muscles to help maintain normal shoulder position.

The following shoulder stretching and strengthening exercises should be performed two to three times a day, with two to three repetitions each time. Gradually increase these exercises to ten times a day with ten repetitions each time. Children under twelve should do only one to two repetitions of these exercises three times a day.

SHOULDER STRETCHING AND STRENGTHENING EXERCISE #1:

The "Shoulder Shrug" Stretch and Strengthener: This exercise will stretch, relax, and loosen your shoulder joints and strengthen your shoulder muscles.

Doctor's prescription:

❑ Do this stretching and strengthening exercise _____ times a day with _____ repetitions each time.

Instructions:

- Stand or sit up straight in a chair that supports your mid back.

- Look straight ahead.

- Keep your head, ears, and chin level.

- Keep your head directly over your shoulders.

- Do not move your head forward, backward, or to the side.

- Keep your arms hanging at your sides.

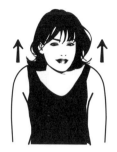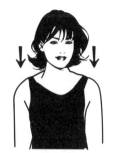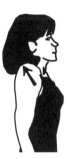

"Shoulder Shrug" Exercise

- Shrug (raise) your shoulders straight upward, as high as they will go.

- Hold this position for eight to ten seconds.

- Slowly return your shoulders down to their normal position.

- Then, depress your shoulders and arms down toward the floor as far as they will go. At the same time, rotate your hands so that your thumbs are facing outward.

- Slowly return your shoulders to their starting position.

- Then, shrug (raise) both shoulders up to ear level and as far backward as possible.

- Hold this position for eight to ten seconds.

- Slowly return your shoulders to their normal position.

- Then, depress your shoulders and arms toward the floor as far as they will go.

- Hold this position for eight to ten seconds.

- Then, slowly return your shoulders to their starting position.

- Limit these motions to your shoulders.

SHOULDER STRETCHING AND STRENGTHENING EXERCISE #2:

Front of Shoulder and Mid Back Stretch and Strengthener: This exercise stretches the shoulders backward and strengthens the shoulder and mid back muscles.

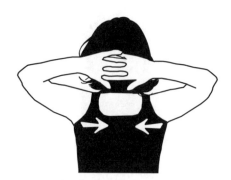

"Shoulder, Mid Back" Stretching/Strengthening Exercise

Doctor's prescription:
☐   Do this stretching and strengthening exercise _____ times a day
with _____ repetitions each time.

Instructions:
- Stand or sit up straight in a chair that supports your mid back.

- Keep your eyes straight ahead with your head and chin level.

- Interlock both hands behind your neck with your elbows straight
out to the side.

- While not allowing your head to be pulled forward, pull your elbows backward and your shoulder blades toward each other as far
as possible.

- Hold this position for eight to ten seconds.

- Then, slowly return to the starting position.

SHOULDER STRETCHING AND STRENGTHENING EXERCISE #3:
The "Shoulder Roll": This stretching and strengthening exercise is
used to stretch, relax, loosen, and strengthen your shoulder, neck, and
upper back muscles.

Doctor's prescription:
☐   Do this stretching and strengthening exercise _____ times a day
with _____ repetitions each time.

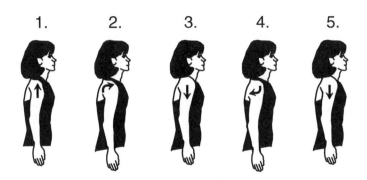

"Shoulder Roll" Exercise

Instructions:

- Sit up straight in a chair that supports your mid back.

- Look straight ahead.

- Keep your head, ears, and chin level.

- Keep you head directly over your shoulders.

- Do not move your head forward, backward, or to the sides.

- Keep your arms hanging at your sides.

- Raise your shoulders straight upward as far as they will go. Hold this position for eight to ten seconds.

- Then, rotate and pull your shoulders forward as far as they will go. Hold this position for eight to ten seconds.

- Then, push your shoulders downward as far as they will go. Hold this position for eight to ten seconds.

- Then, rotate and pull your shoulders down and backward as far as they will go. Hold this position for eight to ten seconds.

- Then, push your shoulders downward as far as they will go. Hold this position for eight to ten seconds.

- Then, slowly return to the starting position.

- Repeat the exercise by reversing the order of these steps.

MID BACK (THORAX) EXERCISES

The following mid back stretching and strengthening exercises should be performed two to three times a day, with two to three repetitions each time. Gradually increase these exercises to ten times a day with ten repetitions each time. Children under twelve should do only one to two repetitions of these exercises three times a day.

Mid Back (Thorax) Stretching Exercises

MID BACK (THORAX) STRETCHING EXERCISE #1:

The "Doorway" Stretch: This exercise stretches the muscles and ligaments of your chest and mid back.

Doctor's prescription:

❏ Do this stretching exercise _____ times a day with _____ repetitions each time.

Instructions:

- Stand in a doorway.

- Place your right forearm against the right door frame and your left forearm against the left door frame.

- Step forward with one knee bent while keeping your back straight.

- Attempt to flatten your mid back and bring your shoulder blades together.

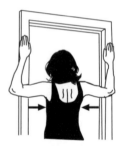

"Doorway Stretch" Exercise

- Then, allow your torso to "sink" forward between your shoulder blades until you feel your shoulder blades being pulled forward against your rib cage.

- Hold this position for eight to ten seconds.

- Then, slowly return to the starting position.

- Do this exercise before performing other exercises for the mid back.

MID BACK (THORAX) STRETCHING EXERCISE #2:

The "Sitting Hitchhiker" Stretch: This exercise stretches the muscles and ligaments of your chest and mid back.

Doctor's prescription:
❑   Do this stretching exercise _____ times a day with _____ repetitions each time.

Instructions:
- Sit on the edge of a chair.

- Place your feet at least twelve inches apart.

- Let your arms hang at your sides.

- Rotate your arms so that your thumbs point outward. Continue rotating your arms until you feel your shoulder blades being pulled together in your mid back.

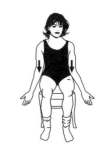

"Sitting Hitchhiker" Stretching Exercise

- Then, drop your shoulders downward as far as they can go.

- Hold this position for eight to ten seconds.

- Then, slowly return to the starting position.

MID BACK (THORAX) STRETCHING EXERCISE #3:

The Sitting Backward Extension Stretch: This exercise stretches the spinal ligaments of your mid back and strengthens your mid back muscles.

Doctor's prescription:
❑   Do this stretching and strengthening exercise _____ times a day with _____ repetitions each time.

Instructions:
- Sit on a chair with your hands on your knees.

- Place your feet at least twelve inches apart.

- Lean forward until your chest touches your knees.

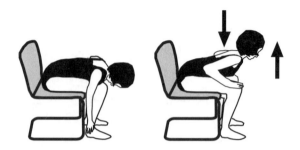

"Sitting Backward Extension" Stretching Exercise

- Slowly bend your head and neck backward while pulling your mid back forward until you feel your spine being pulled downward toward your thighs.

- Then contract (tighten) the muscles of your mid back.

- Hold this position for eight to ten seconds.

- Then, slowly return to the starting position.

Mid Back (Thorax) Strengthening Exercises

MID BACK (THORAX) STRENGTHENING EXERCISE #1:

The "Corner" Push-Up: This stretching and strengthening exercise stretches your chest, pulls your mid back inward, and strengthens your mid back muscles.

Doctor's prescription:

❑   Do this stretching and strengthening exercise _____ times a day with _____ repetitions each time.

Instructions:

- Stand up straight.

- Face one corner of a room.

- Place one hand on each wall at shoulder level and at a width slightly wider than your shoulders.

- Move both feet backward approximately twelve inches. To make this exercise harder, move your feet farther back.

- Bend your knees slightly.

- Bend your elbows and lower your body toward the corner.

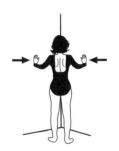

"Corner Push-Up" Exercise

- Attempt to flatten your mid back and bring your shoulder blades together, without letting your lower back sag toward the wall.

- Then, push your body toward the corner until you feel your shoulder blades being pulled forward against your rib cage.

- Hold this position for eight to ten seconds.

- Then, slowly return to the starting position.

MID BACK (THORAX) STRENGTHENING EXERCISE #2:

Backward Bending Mid Back Strengthener: This exercise tightens your mid back and neck muscles. This strengthening exercise is also used to correct a neck that has too much of a forward curve.

Doctor's prescription:
❑ Do this strengthening exercise _____ times a day with _____ repetitions each time

Instructions:
- Stand up straight with your arms stretched out sideways at right angles to your body.

- Rotate your arms and hands so that your thumbs are facing straight upward.

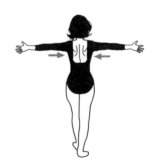

- Then, bring your arms backward one to two inches, or until you feel your shoulder blades being squeezed together.

"Backward-Bending, Mid Back" Strengthening Exercise

- Hold this position for eight to ten seconds.
- Then, slowly return to the starting position.

The neck-aids and neck-appliances described in this chapter can be ordered through your family chiropractor or from the Neck and Back Products store at **www.NeckAndBackProducts.com** or call toll-free **1-800-882-4476.**

Epilogue

The idea of teaching others "how to prevent neck pain" came to me many years ago. As a chiropractor, I relieved the neck and back pain of thousands of patients but was discouraged by the number of patients who came back repeatedly with the very same pain. I realized that something had to be done to help my patients "prevent" their pain from returning.

As their doctor, I knew I couldn't keep my patients' neck pain from returning ... only they could, if they knew how. Thus, following the old adage "an ounce of prevention is worth a pound of cure," I developed a Neck Care class to teach my patients how to change their lifestyles, actions, and environments to eliminate the stresses that could injure or re-injure their necks. The more I taught them, the more they didn't need my care. That should be the objective of any doctor: to cure ... to permanently cure his or her patients.

In this book, I give you the same advice that helped my patients.

Only you can prevent having pain in your neck. As a doctor and author, I can teach you how. This book tells you what you can do, as well as what you shouldn't do, to prevent neck pain. You'll first learn about making certain changes in your sleeping posture and about properly supporting your neck in bed. Then you'll learn how to achieve a neck-friendly environment through the use of specific ergonomic modifications. Lastly, you will learn how to strengthen your neck muscles by following a simple stretching and exercise program. This is your opportunity to live a life free of neck pain (barring the occurrence of accidental injury).

This book has been a joy for me to write ... it is an extension of who I am and what I love to do ... a doctor helping patients get well. I welcome your comments and suggestions. Please write me at *DrPete@NeckPainNeckPain.com.* I would love to hear from you.

APPENDIX: RESOURCES

Neck and Back Care Products

Many of the neck-aids and neck-appliances described in this book are special-care items that may be difficult to find in your area. As a convenience, items mentioned in this book may be purchased through your family chiropractor or ordered from the Neck and Back Products store at *www.NeckAndBackProducts.com* or by calling 1-800-882-4476.*

AUTOMOTIVE PRODUCTS

100   Lumbar Support for Automobiles
101   Add-On Headrests
102   Rearview Radar Device
103   Vibration Dampening Cushion
104   Plastic Support Seat
105   Liquid-Filled Pillow (Cushion)
106   Car Seat Riser Cushion
107   Wedge-Shaped Cushion
108   "Fisheye" Mirror
109   Panoramic Rearview Mirror
110   Add-On Console
111   Add-On Padded Armrest
112   Seat Belt Adjuster
486   Additional Automotive Support Handle

BABY PRODUCTS

200   Baby Sling
201   Backpack Baby Carrier
202   Front Baby Carrier
203   Child Safety Seat
204   Circular Head and Neck Support
205   Child Booster Seat

---

*The reader accepts sole liability for determining whether items and/or ideas contained in this book are appropriate for the reader.

BATHROOM PRODUCTS

450 Fog-Free Mirror

451 Non-Skid Bathroom Mat

452 Long-Handled Scrub Brush

453 Triangular Shower Shelves

454 Shower Shelves that Attach to Showerhead

455 Shower Shelves on a Pole

456 Shower Stool

457 Raised Foot Receptacle

458 Curved Shower Rod

459 Hair Dryer Stand

460 Adjustable Mirror

461 Wall Mirror

462 Magnifying Mirror

463 Free-Standing Toilet Paper Holder

464 Over-the-Sink Shelf

480 Adjustable Wall Mirror

481 Mirror on a Stand

482 Hose Attachment

483 Walk-In Bathtub

BEDROOM PRODUCTS

401 Bed Lounger

402 Reading Pillow

403 Tilting Bed Tray

408 Cervical Contour Pillow

409 Cervical Roll

410 Night Roll

411 Knee Elevator Pillow

412 Positioning Wedge

413 Stomach Sleeping Pillow

414 Kapok Pillow

415 Visco-Elastic (Memory Foam) Pillow

416 Water Pillow

417 Air Pillow

418 Air Pillow with Multiple Bladders

419 Side-Sleeper Pillow
420 Travel Pillow
421 Contoured Knee Pillow
422 Visco-Elastic (Memory-Foam) Mattress
423 Multi-Zone Mattress & Springs
424 Inner Spring Mattress & Springs
425 Air Mattress
426 Water Bed
427 Crescent-Shaped Pillow

BODY SUPPORT PRODUCTS
702 Shoe Orthotics
700 Adjustable Lumbar Support

CLOSET PRODUCTS
477 Hanging Shoe Bag/Rack
478 Hanging Jewelry Organizer
479 Motorized Tie Organizer

COMPUTER PRODUCTS
510 Articulating Arm for Telephone
511 Keyboard Tray
512 Document Holder
513 Articulating Arm for Computer Monitor
515 Computer Riser
516 Anti-Glare Computer Monitor Hood
517 Non-Glare Computer Light
518 Wall Mount Computer Support
519 Articulating Arm for Document Holder
520 Free-Standing Paper Holder
521 Wireless Computer Keyboard
522 Ergonomic Keyboard
523 Padded Wrist Support
524 Gel-Filled Wrist Support
525 Raised Document Holder

DRESSING PRODUCTS

446 Long-Handled Shoe Horn
447 Ergonomically Correct Purse
448 Ergonomically Correct Briefcase
449 Ergonomically Correct Backpack
465 Rolling Backpack

EXERCISE PRODUCTS

300 Posture Pulley
301 Neck Strengthening Device

FURNITURE

404 Natural Daylight Lamp
406 Step Stool
445 Footrest
466 Clothes & Hat Rack
471 Special Support Board
475 Adjustable Computer Desk
484 Reclining Chaise Lounge
485 Wooden or Plastic Blocks
701 Wedge-Shaped Pillow

INSIDE HOME MAINTENANCE PRODUCTS

407 Long-Handled Reaching Stick
428 Robotic Vacuum Cleaner
429 Ergonomic Push Broom
430 Combination Motorized Broom and Dust Pan
431 Ergonomic Mop
432 Robotic Floor Washer

KITCHEN PRODUCTS

467 Ergonomic Knives
468 Horizontal Utensil Rack
469 Ergonomic Pots & Pans
470 Ergonomic Garbage Pail

OFFICE PRODUCTS

501   Speakerphone
503   Slantboard
504   Ergonomically Correct Desk
505   Large Document Holder
506   Desk Shelf
507   Ergonomically Adjustable Chair
508   Hands-Free Headset
509   Built-Up Phone Handle
514   Bookstand
526   Anti-Fatigue Rubber Mat
700   Adjustable Lumbar Support

OUTSIDE HOME MAINTENANCE PRODUCTS

433   Ergonomic Long-Handled Rake
434   Ergonomic Hoe
435   Portable Garden Seat
436   Rolling Garden Seat
437   Ergonomic Shovel
438   Wheelbarrow with Large Wheels
439   Automatic Hose Rewinder
440   Coiled Garden Hose
441   Rolling Tool Organizer/Carrier
442   Snow Shovel Push Blade with Wheels
443   Snow Scoop
444   Push Snow Shovel

READING PRODUCTS

400   Side-Reading Slantboard
405   Book Light
472   Narrow Beam Reading Light
473   Adjustable Reading Table
474   Adjustable Magnifying Device

TRAVEL PRODUCTS

800   Collapsible Luggage Carrier with Wheels
801   Inflatable Travel Pillow

Doctor Locator

I would like to acknowledge the following "neck specialist" chiropractors for their fine work, professional research, and patient care instructions that were the basis for this book. I extend my sincere appreciation to these caring D.C.s on behalf of myself and the thousands of neck pain sufferers who will use this book to achieve a life free of neck pain.

—Dr. Peter G. Fernandez

CONTRIBUTING AUTHORS

ALABAMA
BIRMINGHAM, AL 35216
DR. MARK N. BERRY
1442 MONTGOMERY HWY 31
205-994-1993
drberrychiro@yahoo.com
www.berrychiro.com

GADSDEN, AL 35901
DR. ROYCE H. JONES
1615 RAINBOW DR.
256-547-1603
drroycejones@ainweb.net

MOBILE, AL 36609
DR. ANTHONY W. VICHETO
1956 "H" S. UNIVERSITY BLVD.
251-665-9898
drvicheto@aol.com
www.vichetochiro.com

MOBILE, AL 36695

> DR. JEFF S. WOODRUFF
> 1516 SCHILLINGER RD. SOUTH
> 251-635-1224
> dcin2000@yahoo.com
> www.jeffwoodruff.com

VESTAVIA HILLS, AL 35216

> DR. MARK N. BERRY
> 1442 MONTGOMERY HWY 31
> 205-994-1993
> drberrychiro@yahoo.com
> www.berrychiro.com

ALASKA

JUNEAU, AK 99801

> DR. GORDON L. SHEPRO
> ADVANCE CHIROPRACTIC
> 2243 N. JORDAN AVE.
> 907-790-3371
> allchiro@alaska.com
> www.allchiro.net

ARIZONA

PHOENIX, AZ 85014

> ROBERT LEE GEAR, JR., D.C., N.M.D.
> 3543 N. 7TH ST.
> 602-263-8484
> naturopathicphy@pol.net
> www.comprehensive.ws

CALIFORNIA
CHICO, CA 95926
> DR. LARRY E. MASULA
> 250 VALLOMBROSA, STE. 450
> 530-342-6441
> mazudoc@sbcglobal.net

SAN RAFAEL, CA 94901
> DR. JONATHAN HYSLOP
> 806 FOURTH ST.
> 415-456-3232
> drjonathanhyslop@mac.com
> www.hyslopchiropractic.com

SOUTH LAKE TAHOE, CA 96150
> DR. DAVID BORGES
> 2074 LAKE TAHOE BLVD., STE. 5
> 530-544-5800
> coachdbdc@yahoo.com
> www.borgeschiro.com

> DR. KAREN M. BORGES
> 2074 LAKE TAHOE BLVD., STE. 5
> 530-544-5800
> borges01@sbcglobal.net
> www.borgeschiro.com

TORRANCE, CA 90505
> DR. DAVID R. DAUER
> 22930 HAWTHORNE BLVD.
> 310-378-9990
> holisticdoctorgroup@yahoo.com
> www.drdauer.com

CONNECTICUT
GROTON, CT 06340
DR. JOSEPH A. MASCARO
565 LONG HILL RD.
860-448-1442
joemascaro@aol.com
www.advancedbackandneck.com

NORWALK, CT 06851
DR. BRENDA. SLOVIN
205 MAIN AVE.
203-840-0000
contact@headache-neck-pain-relief.com;
www.headache-neck-pain-relief.com

DR. ERIK SLOVIN
205 MAIN AVE.
203-840-0000
contact@headache-neck-pain-relief.com;
www.headache-neck-pain-relief.com

FLORIDA
APOLLO BEACH, FL 33572
DR. STEPHEN D. MURRAY
100 FRANDORSON CIR., STE. 101
813-641-3333
apollobeachchiro@aol.com
www.apollobeachchiro.com

BELLEAIR BLUFFS, FL 33770
DR. ROBERT A. FADY
490 N. INDIAN ROCKS RD., STE. B
727-585-4300
fadyr@msn.com

DELRAY BEACH, FL 33445
DR. RYAN S. ALTER
4205 W. ATLANTIC AVE., STE. 102
561-819-2225
DrAlter@aol.com
www.alterchiropractic.com

FORT LAUDERDALE, FL 33312
DR. LAURENCE J. BURCH
3267 W. DAVIE BLVD.
954-587-5700
drlarryburch@aol.com
www.drburchpaincenter.com

JACKSONVILLE, FL 32218
DR. SCOTT M. MEIDE
2255 DUNN AVE., STE. 201
904-696-1929
jsicenter@bellsouth.net

LADY LAKE, FL 32159
DR. JAMES A. SCOTT
13767 U.S. HWY 441
352-430-1890
dr.jamesscott@earthlink.net
www.scott-chiropractic.com

MIAMI, FL
DR. DIANA FINLEY
305-336-8335
dlf826@yahoo.com
www.drdianafinley.com

OCALA, FL 34471

DR. DAVID N. KREINBROOK
27 S.E. 11TH AVE.
352-732-5590
drkreinbrook@yahoo.com
www.drkreinbrook.com

OCALA, FL 34474

DR. GARY P. STEPHENS
3101 S.W. 34 AVE., STE. 202
352-622-4555
yourchiro1@earthlink.net
www.yourchiro.net

PALM HARBOR, FL 34683

DR. KEVIN M. GALLAGHER
550 ALT 19 NORTH
727-789-0800
doctorg@tampabay.rr.com

PONTE VEDRA BEACH, FL 32082

DR. R.G. PACKO
252 SOLANA RD.
904-285-2243
docpacko@aol.com
www.votedbestdoctor.com

ST. PETERSBURG, FL 33702

DR. G. STANFORD PIERCE, SR.
2201 62ND AVE. NORTH
727-528-8700
atlasortho@aol.com
www.advancedorthogonal.com

ST. PETERSBURG, FL 33702 (Cont'd)
DR. G. STANFORD PIERCE, JR.
2201 62ND AVE. NORTH
727-528-8700
gpierce@tampabay.rr.com
www.advancedorthogonal.com

ST. PETERSBURG, FL 33703
DR. DIANNE M. FERNANDEZ
4800 4TH ST. NORTH
727-528-1133
drdianne@tampabay.rr.com
www.drdiannedc.com

ST. PETERSBURG, FL 33704
DR. RAYMOND P. FERNANDEZ
3326 9TH ST. NORTH
727-822-3604
alexchrissara@msn.com

ST. PETERSBURG, FL 33705
DR. D. PETER MOSHER
6205 DR. MLK JR. ST. SOUTH
727-864-1701
dpetermosher@yahoo.com
www.mosherchiropractic.com

TALLAHASSEE, FL 32301
DR. WILLIAM D. M. ATKINSON, III
2619 BLAIR STONE RD.
850-656-2200
nexnbax1@comcast.net
www.fiorinichiropractic.com

DR. DENNIS G. FIORINI
2619 BLAIR STONE RD.
850-656-2200
spinedoc@nettally.com
www.fiorinichiropractic.com

THE VILLAGES, FL 32162

DR. JASON E. DAVIS

DAVIS CLINIC OF CHIROPRACTIC, INC.

1950 LAUREL MANOR DR., STE. 124

352-430-2121

jasondavisdc@comcast.net

www.davisclinic.org

WINTER HAVEN, FL 33880

DR. GARY W. NEWBERRY

1619 6TH ST. S.E.

863-293-3893

dr.newberry@thenewberryclinic.com

GEORGIA

AUGUSTA, GA 30906

DR. SCOTT J. PIDCOCK

3009 PEACH ORCHARD RD.

706-798-8980

skpid@aol.com

CHAMBLEE, GA 30341

DR. MICHAEL B. WAX

5464 PEACHTREE INDUSTRIAL BLVD.

770-454-8300

michaelwax@bellsouth.net

FAYETTEVILLE, GA 30214

DR. LINDA H. KATZ

126 NEW HOPE RD.

770-461-2225

fayettechiro@mindspring.com

www.fayettechiropractic.com

DR. VINCE VELLUCCI

185 GEORGIA AVE. EAST

770-461-0055

GAINESVILLE, GA 30501

DR. MARY E. WATKINS
961 GREEN ST. N.E.
770-534-0656
jsartor@charter.net
www.watkinschiropractic.com

PERRY, GA 31069

DR. BRIAN GILLIS
PERRY CHIROPRACTIC HEALTH CENTER
1207 HOUSTON LAKE DR., STE. C
478-987-9666
drbgillis@yahoo.com
www.perrychiropractichealthcenter.com

SAVANNAH, GA 31404

DR. BART WETHERINGTON
5602 WATERS AVE., STE. B
912-351-0005
drwetherington@bellsouth.net;
www.wetheringtonchiropractic.com

TUCKER, GA 30084

DR. JOEL E. MARGOLIES
4910 LAVISTA RD.
770-491-3639
joel3639@aol.com
www.chirosmart.net

ILLINOIS

BELLEVILLE, IL 62226

DR. KATHLEEN M. ROCHE
3915 W. MAIN
618-234-1455
drkathy4401@peaknet.net
www.gotbackpain.net

BOLINGBROOK, IL 60440

>DR. ANN MARIE F. RUSSELL
>477 BOLINGBROOK DR.
>630-759-4949
>drrussell4949@sbcglobal.net

GALESBURG, IL 61401

>DR. JEFFREY L. HAYDEN
>1174 N. SEMINARY ST.
>309-344-4988
>atlasharvard@netscape.net
>www.doctorhayden.com

GRANITE CITY, IL 62040

>DR. LAWRENCE A. SHIPLEY
>2502 PONTOON RD.
>618-931-2001
>plship@charter.net
>www.shipleychiropractic.com

SCHAUMBURG, IL 60193

>DR. HIROYA NAKAMURA
>655 S. ROSELLE RD.
>847-891-1112
>hiroya_n@hotmail.com
>www.nakamurachiropractic.topchiro.com

INDIANA
EVANSVILLE, IN 47715

>DR. BENJAMIN B. DICKINSON
>3101 N. GREEN RIVER RD., STE. 110
>812-491-7777
>drdickinson@earthlink.net
>www.dickinsonchiropractic.com

EVANSVILLE, IN 47715 (Cont'd)
DR. DEANA REHMEL
3101 N. GREEN RIVER RD., STE. 110
812-491-7777
drrehmel@earthlink.net
www.dickinsonchiropractic.com

RENSSELAER, IN 47978
DR. STEVE L. JENNINGS
101 N. AUSTIN AVE.
219-866-7164
Jennings@midwaynet.net

KENTUCKY
FAIRDALE, KY 40118
DR. MOSEN R. KHANI
10701 W. MANSLICK RD.
502-367-2112
fixbax@bellsouth.net

LEXINGTON, KY 40503
DR. JEFFREY W. STINSON
1529 NICHOLASVILLE RD.
859-276-1123
drstinson@insightbb.com
www.drjeffreystinson.com

MAYFIELD, KY 42066
DANIEL R. FARR, D.C.
319 S 9TH ST.
270-251-0907
primarycare101@bellsouth.net

LOUISIANA
MONROE, LA 71201
> DR. BRIAN D. COLEMAN
> 2501 FERRAND ST.
> 318-388-2215
> admin@colemanchiropractic.net
> www.colemanchiropractic.net

MAINE
AUBURN, ME 04210
> DR. GERALD A. NADEAU
> 336 CENTER ST.
> 207-777-1104
> drnadeau@gwi.net
> www.drganadeau.com

MARYLAND
GLEN BURNIE, MD 21061
> DR. ADAM M. BRENNER
> 7450 BALTIMORE ANNAPOLIS BLVD.
> 410-424-2266
> ambrenner@hotmail.com

SILVER SPRING, MD 20910
> DR. MOHAMMAD YOUSEFI
> 9200 COLESVILLE RD.
> 301-585-3200
> yousefichiropractic@yahoo.com
> www.yousefichiropractic.com

MASSACHUSETTS
NORTHAMPTON, MA 01060
> DR. KIMBERLY LANGE
> 141 DAMON RD.
> 413-582-9889
> drlange@langechiropractic.com
> www.langechiropractic.com

MINNESOTA
MANKATO, MN 56001
> DR. RICHARD A. SAGGAU
> 83 NAVAHO AVE., STE. 26
> 507-625-9060
> rasaggau@hickorytech.net
> www.drsaggau.com

MINNEAPOLIS, MN 55402
> DR. GARY T. MILLER
> 501 MARQUETTE AVE., STE. 170
> 612-870-1500
> ohwdc@msn.com
> www.chiromeridian.com

ST. CLOUD, MN 56303
> DR. DENNIS A. WOGGON
> ST. CLOUD CHIROPRACTIC CLINIC PA
> 437 N. 33RD AVE.
> 320-252-5599
> dwoggon@aol.com
> www.clear-institute.com

MISSISSIPPI
CLINTON, MS 39056
> DR. ALAN N. RATHBURN
> 612 HIGHWAY 80 EAST
> 601-924-4647
> arathb1745@aol.com

RIDGELAND, MS 39157
> DR. LEO C. HUDDLESTON
> 6500 OLD CANTON RD.
> 601-956-0010
> drnatrl@xspedius.net

MISSOURI
GLADSTONE, MO 64118

DR. FRANK R. CARELLA
180 N.E. 72ND ST.
816-436-4369
doctorcare@netscape.com
www.carellachiropractic.com

NEVADA
NORTH LAS VEGAS, NV 89031

DR. JOSEPH D. STEWART
5514 CAMINO AL NORTE, STE. A-2
702-531-3400
joechiropractor@earthlink.net
www.northlasvegaspainrelief.com

NEW JERSEY
CINNAMINSON, NJ 08077

DR. JOHN E. SANDOZ
1104 RT. 130, STE. Q
856-829-8194
jsandoz295017@comcast.net
www.sandozchiropractic.com

COLUMBUS, NJ 08022

DR. DAVID W. IKEDA
23659 COLUMBUS RD., STE. 2A
609-298-7700
dikeda@comcast.net

FORT LEE, NJ 07024

DR. MIKA ISHITANI
1515 PALISADES AVE.
201-302-9993
info@ishitanichiropractic.com
www.ishitanichiropractic.com

GIBBSTOWN, NJ 08027

DR. BLAISE K. GLODOWSKI, Ground Zero Volunteer
360 E. BROAD ST.
856-423-3899
drhealth@snip.net
www.gibbstownchiropractic.com

NEWARK, NJ 07105

DR. PAULO J. PEREIRA
40 FERRY ST. (Near Penn Station)
973-465-1500
pereiradc@yahoo.com
www.drpereira.com

NORTH BERGEN, NJ 07047

DR. ALEX M. HERNANDEZ
8325 KENNEDY BLVD.
201-861-2025
dr_alexh@verizon.net
www.dralexhernandez.com

NORTH PLAINFIELD, NJ 07060

DR. PAUL F. LYONS
50 GREENBROOK RD.
908-755-2111

NEW YORK
DUTCHESS COUNTY, NY

DR. ANDREA PAPORTO
678-778-6553
drpaporto@aol.com
www.paportochiropractic.com

STATEN ISLAND, NY 10312
DR. ROBERT M. BROWNE
4634 AMBOY RD.
718-356-8438
wecarechiro@aol.com
www.wecarechiro.com

NORTH CAROLINA
ASHEVILLE, NC 28801
DR. M. JAROD DOSTER
DR. TANYA E. DOSTER
828-236-2200
ziggy3430@yahoo.com
www.drdoster.com

CHARLOTTE, NC 28209
DR. MARCUS O. SCHUSTER
4832 PARK RD., STE. J
704-561-9494
drschuster@schusterchiropractic.com
www.schusterchiropractic.com

GOLDSBORO, NC 27534
DR. WAYNE D. PALMER
1401 N. BERKELEY BLVD., STE. H
919-778-7871
waynechirocenter@bellsouth.net

MAYODAN, NC 27027
DR. KEITH H. LINEBERRY
901 S. AYERSVILLE RD.
336-548-2225
Khlineberry@yahoo.com

WINSTON-SALEM, NC
DR. M. JAROD DOSTER
DR. TANYA E. DOSTER
828-236-2200
ziggy3430@yahoo.com
www.drdoster.com

OHIO
MEDINA, OH 44256-2666
DR. CARL V. BRUNELLO
600 E. SMITH RD., STE. A
330-725-4500
brunello9@hotmail.com

POWELL, OH 43065
DR. JOHN A. ELLWOOD
128 E. OLENTANGY ST.
614-985-3383
drjohnellwood@yahoo.com
www.headandneckclinic.com

REYNOLDSBURG, OH 43068
DR. JAMES E. HICKS
6400 E. MAIN ST.
614-864-1611
drjhicks1000@aol.com
www.doctorhicks.com

OKLAHOMA
MADILL, OK 73446
DR. JAMES W. TALLEY
411 N. FIRST ST.
580-795-2269
jamestalleydc@sbcglobal.net
www.doctortalley.com

TULSA, OK 74136
DR. BRAD M. HAYES
6717 S. YALE AVE., STE. 110
918-492-0087
dcbrad1@aol.com
www.chiropractordrs.com

PENNSYLVANIA
ALLENTOWN, PA 18101
DR. GEORGE L. JENKINS
43 N. 4TH ST.
P.O. BOX 1485
484-788-0190
drjenkins@joust.net

HUNTINGTON VALLEY, PA 19006
DR. LEN S. SCHWARTZ
3983 MANN RD.
866-655-8502
Chiropower1@comcast.net
www.askdoctorlen.com

KINGSTON, PA 18704
DR. MALCOLM L. CONWAY
575 PIERCE ST., STE. 102
570-287-7070
drc@docconway.com
www.conwayclinic.com

LANGHORNE, PA 19047
DR. DAVID R. TUCKER
198 N. PINE ST.
215-750-8006
healthyspines@hotmail.com

LEBANON, PA 17042
> DR. GEORGE L. JENKINS
> 518 S. 8TH ST.
> 717-273-5959
> drjenkins@joust.net

SEWICKLEY, PA 15143
> DR. WILLIAM N. CANNISTER
> 201 OHIO RIVER BLVD.
> 412-741-2646

SOUTH CAROLINA
PENDLETON, SC 29670
> DR. RICHARD LOHR
> 7611 HWY. 76, STE. C
> 864-646-2200
> rich.lohr@comcast.net

SUMMERVILLE, SC 29483
> DR. DREW K. MCPHAIL
> 215 E. 5TH NORTH ST.
> 843-873-2225
> drewkmcphail@yahoo.com
> www.mcphailchiropractic.com

TENNESSEE
DUNLAP, TN 37327
> MONTY C. LONG, D.C.
> LONG FAMILY CHIROPRACTIC, INC.
> 86 FRONTAGE RD.
> P.O. BOX 936
> 423-949-5599
> longchiro@bledsoe.net
> www.drlong.net

MONTEAGLE, TN 37356
DR. VICTOR T. PALFFY
16 E. MAIN ST.
P.O. BOX 545
931-924-3474
palffychiro@blomand.net
www.drvictortpalffy.com

TEXAS
ARLINGTON, TX 76016
DR. KEVIN L. TOMSIC
7108 ROYAL GATES DR.
214-727-1971
ktmddc@hotmail.com

ATHENS, TX 75751
DR. DANA J. SANTELLI
890 W. CORSICANA ST.
903-677-1936
djs5386@cox-internet.com

AUSTIN, TX 78741
DR. DON A. SALYER
2410 E. RIVERSIDE DR., STE. H-11
512-442-4357
capitalchiropracticdrsalyer@yahoo.com
www.capitalchiropractic.com

COPPELL, TX 75019
DR. RON H. CARPENTER
454 PHILLIPS
972-462-8282
469-360-2655
coppellchiro@yahoo.com
www.coppellchiro.com

DENTON, TX 76201
DR. KARL JAWHARI
1010 N. ELM, STE. C
940-566-6645
drjawhari@aol.com
www.elmstreetchiro.com

EL PASO, TX 79924
DR. CARLOS R. RODRIGUEZ
5140 FAIRBANKS, STE. 3
915-757-6600
carlosrelpaso@aol.com
www.rodriguez-chiro-acu.com

FORT WORTH, TX 76140-2358
DR. MICHAEL GRAY
6801 RUFE SNOW DR., STE. 110
817-656-1615
amg7@hotmail.com
www.texashealthquest.com

GALVESTON, TX 77551
DR. DONNA S. SANDERS
2115 61ST ST., STE. 101
409-740-7977
chirosan1@sbcglobal.net

IRVING, TX 75063
DR. KELLY LEE CATO
214-497-0262
kcato@parkercc.edu

KELLER, TX 76248
DR. HOWARD C. GLANS
INTEGRATED SPINAL DECOMPRESSION CENTER, P.A.
426 KELLER PKWY., STE. 500
817-798-4226
drglans@charter.net
www.backinstep.net

PORT ISABEL, TX 78578
DR. KENNETH J. COPELAND
215 QUEEN ISABELLA BLVD.
956-943-9355
dr@lighthouse.com
www.lighthousechiropractic.com

SUGARLAND, TX 77478
DR. STEPHEN A. HARRIS
3425 HWY 6, STE. 101
281-980-1050
sharris8@flash.net
www.harrisneckandback.com

UTAH
OREM, UT 84058
DR. S. R. RUTKOWSKI
361 E. UNIVERSITY PKWY.
801-224-3413
s.r.rutkowski@att.net

VIRGINIA
ALEXANDRIA, VA 22314
DR. ROBERT M. KNAPP
2817 DUKE ST.
703-823-2201
unonemo@yahoo.com
www.aachiropractic.com

CHESAPEAKE, VA 23322
DR. JOSH D. REED
1464 MT. PLEASANT RD., STE. 13
757-546-8888
drreed@drjoshreed.com
www.drjoshreed.com

LYNCHBURG, VA 24502

DR. DANIEL M. JARVIS
7204 TIMBERLAKE RD.
434-239-9993
drdanjarvis@drdanjarvis.com
www.drdanjarvis.com

DR. ROB S. JARVIS
5521 FORT AVE.
434-239-0023
rjarvis@lacil.org
www.lynchburgsaves.com

VIRGINIA BEACH, VA 23451

DR. JULIA A. STICKELL
936 GENERAL BOOTH BLVD., STE. C
757-422-2232

WASHINGTON

BATTLE GROUND, WA 98604

DR. THOMAS J. OPDAHL
201 N. PARKWAY AVE., STE. 101
360-666-6001
opdahldc@hotmail.com
www.battlegroundchiropractic.com

HOQUIAM, WA 98550

DR. MARK R. VAN HEMERT
2223 SIMPSON AVE.
360-533-6400
hemert@techline.com

CANADA

ONTARIO
PORT COLBORNE, ONT L3K-6A6

DR. DAVID G. SALANKI
258 KILLALY ST. WEST
905-835-1303
dsalanki@chiropracticassociates.com
www.chiropracticassociates.com

QUEBEC
BROMONT, QUE J2L-1A9

DR. GILLES H. BRUNELLE
P.O. BOX 188
450-531-9373
drgbrunelle@hotmail.com

Index

How to Engage the Author

Dr. Peter G. Fernandez, D.C.
Chiropractic Marketing & Development
Speaking – Seminars – Coaching – Consulting

Dr. Peter G. Fernandez
10733 57th Ave. N.
Seminole, FL 33772

Phone: 800–882–4476
Fax: 727–392–0489

www.NeckPainNeckPain.com
DrPete@NeckPainNeckPain.com